IARC MONOGRAPHS ON THE

EVALUATION OF THE CARCINOGENIC RISK

OF CHEMICALS TO HUMANS

Some Non-Nutritive Sweetening Agents

Volume 22

This publication represents the views and expert opinions
of an IARC Working Group on the
Evaluation of the Carcinogenic Risk of Chemicals to Humans
which met in Lyon,
21-27 March 1979

March 1980

INTERNATIONAL AGENCY FOR RESEARCH ON CANCER

IARC MONOGRAPHS

In 1971, the International Agency for Research on Cancer (IARC) initiated a programme on the evaluation of the carcinogenic risk of chemicals to humans involving the production of critically evaluated monographs on individual chemicals.

The objective of the programme is to elaborate and publish in the form of monographs critical reviews of data on carcinogenicity for groups of chemicals to which humans are known to be exposed, to evaluate these data in terms of human risk with the help of international working groups of experts in chemical carcinogenesis and related fields, and to indicate where additional research efforts are needed.

International Agency for Research on Cancer 1980

ISBN 92 832 1222 3

PRINTED IN SWITZERLAND

CONTENTS

IARC WORKING GROUP ON THE EVALUATION OF THE CARCINOGENIC RISK OF CHEMICALS TO HUMANS:

SOME NON-NUTRITIVE SWEETENING AGENTS

Lyon, 21-27 March 1979

Members[1]

J. Althoff, Abteilung für Experimentelle Pathologie, Medizinische Hochschule Hannover, Karl-Wiechert-Allee 9, 3000 Hannover 6, Federal Republic of Germany

E. Boyland, London School of Hygiene and Tropical Medicine, Keppel Street, London WC1E 7HT, UK

N.E. Breslow, Department of Biostatistics, SC-32, University of Washington, Seattle, Washington 98195, USA

G.T. Bryan, Professor, Human Oncology, Department of Human Oncology, Wisconsin Clinical Cancer Center, University of Wisconsin, 600 Highland Avenue, Madison, Wisconsin 53792, USA

E. Farber, Professor and Chairman, Department of Pathology, The University of Toronto, Banting Institute, 100 College Street, Toronto, Ontario M5G 1L5, Canada (*Chairman*)

R.M. Hicks, Reader in Experimental Pathology, The School of Pathology, The Middlesex Hospital Medical School, Riding House Street, London W1P 7LD, UK

M.C. Hollstein, Department of Biochemistry, The University of California, Berkeley, California 94720, USA

A.B. Miller, Director, Epidemiology Unit NCIC, Faculty of Medicine, McMurrich Building, University of Toronto, Toronto, Ontario M5S 1A8, Canada

[1] Unable to attend: Representative from the US Manufacturing Chemists Association: Dr G. Levinskas, Monsanto Company, 800 N. Lindbergh Boulevard, St Louis, Missouri 63166, USA

6

I.C. Munro, Chief, Toxicology Research Division, Health and Welfare Canada, Health Protection Branch, Tunney's Pasture, Ottawa, Ontario K1A 0L2, Canada

D. Neubert, Institut für Toxikologie und Embryonal-Pharmakologie der Freien Universität Berlin, Garystrasse 9, 1000 Berlin 33, Federal Republic of Germany

C. Schlatter, Institut für Toxikologie der Eidgenössischen Technischen Hochschule und der Universität Zürich, Schorenstrasse 16, 8603 Schwerzenbach bei Zürich, Switzerland (*Vice-Chairman*)

B. Teichmann, Department of Chemical Carcinogenesis, Zentralinstitut für Krebsforschung, Akademie der Wissenschaften der DDR, Lindenberger Weg 80, 1115 Berlin-Buch, German Democratic Republic

H.A. Tyroler, Professor of Epidemiology, Department of Epidemiology, The School of Public Health, The University of North Carolina, Rosenau Hall 201 H, Chapel Hill, North Carolina 27514, USA

N. Wald, ICRF Cancer Epidemiology and Clinical Trials Unit, University of Oxford, Department of the Regius Professor of Medicine, Radcliffe Infirmary, Oxford OX2 6HE, UK

Representative from the US National Cancer Institute

T.P. Cameron, Assistant Scientific Coordinator for Environmental Cancer, Division of Cancer Cause and Prevention, National Cancer Institute, Landow Building, Bethesda, Maryland 20014, USA

Representative from SRI International

K.E. McCaleb, Director, Chemical-Environmental Program, Chemical Industries Center, SRI International, 333 Ravenswood Avenue, Menlo Park, California 94025, USA (*Rapporteur sections 2.1 and 2.2*)

Representative from the Commission of the European Communities

M-T. van der Venne, Commission of the European Communities, Health and Safety Directorate, Batiment Jean Monnet, Plateau du Kirchberg, Luxembourg, Great Duchy of Luxembourg

Representative from the World Health Organization

G. Vettorazzi, Environmental Health Criteria and Standards (Food Safety), Division of Environmental Health, World Health Organization, 1211 Geneva 27, Switzerland

Observers

W. Grunow, Abteilung für Toxikologie, Bundesgesundheitsamt, Thielallee 88/92, 1 Berlin 33 - Postfach, Federal Republic of Germany

J. Hooson, British Industrial Biological Research Association, Woodmansterne Road, Carshalton, Surrey SM5 4DS, UK

Secretariat

C. Agthe, Director's Office
R. Althouse[1], Unit of Chemical Carcinogenesis
H. Bartsch, Unit of Chemical Carcinogenesis (*Rapporteur section 3.2*)
J.A. Cooper[2], Unit of Epidemiology and Biostatistics (*Co-rapporteur section 3.3*)
J. Esteve, Unit of Epidemiology and Biostatistics
M. Friesen, Unit of Environmental Carcinogens
L. Griciute, Chief, Unit of Environmental Carcinogens
J.E. Huff[3], Unit of Chemical Carcinogenesis (*Co-secretary*)

[1] Present address: University of Oxford, Department of the Regius Professor of Medicine, Radcliffe Infirmary, Oxford OX2 6HE, UK

[2] Present address: Deputy Associate Director, Carcinogenesis Program, Division of Cancer Cause and Treatment, National Cancer Institute, Bethesda, Md 20014, USA

[3] Present address: National Institute of Environmental Health Sciences, P.O. Box 12233, Research Triangle Park, North Carolina 27709, USA

D. Mietton, Unit of Chemical Carcinogenesis (*Library assistant*)

R. Montesano, Unit of Chemical Carcinogenesis (*Rapporteur section 3.1*)

C.S. Muir, Chief, Unit of Epidemiology and Biostatistics

C. Partensky, Unit of Chemical Carcinogenesis (*Technical editor*)

I. Peterschmitt, Unit of Chemical Carcinogenesis, WHO, Geneva (*Bibliographic researcher*)

V. Ponomarkov[1], Unit of Chemical Carcinogenesis

R. Saracci, Unit of Epidemiology and Biostatistics (*Co-rapporteur section 3.3*)

L. Tomatis, Chief, Unit of Chemical Carcinogenesis (*Head of the Programme*)

E.A. Walker, Unit of Environmental Carcinogens (*Rapporteur sections 1 and 2.3*)

E. Ward, Chârost, France (*Editor*)

J.D. Wilbourn, Unit of Chemical Carcinogenesis (*Co-secretary*)

H. Yamasaki, Unit of Chemical Carcinogenesis

Secretarial assistance

A.V. Anderson

M.-J. Ghess

R. Johnson

J. Smith

[1] Present address: Laboratory of Comparative Oncology, Cancer Research Center, USSR Academy of Medical Sciences, Kashirskoye Shosse 6, Moscow 115478, USSR

NOTE TO THE READER

The term 'carcinogenic risk' in the *IARC Monograph* series is taken to mean the probability that exposure to the chemical will lead to cancer in humans.

Inclusion of a chemical in the monographs does not imply that it is a carcinogen, only that the published data have been examined. Equally, the fact that a chemical has not yet been evaluated in a monograph does not mean that it is not carcinogenic.

Anyone who is aware of published data that may alter the evaluation of the carcinogenic risk of a chemical for humans is encouraged to make this information available to the Division of Chemical and Biological Carcinogenesis, International Agency for Research on Cancer, Lyon, France, in order that the chemical may be considered for re-evaluation by a future Working Group.

Although every effort is made to prepare the monographs as accurately as possible, mistakes may occur. Readers are requested to communicate any errors to the Division of Chemical and Biological Carcinogenesis, so that corrections can be reported in future volumes.

IARC MONOGRAPH PROGRAMME ON THE EVALUATION OF THE CARCINOGENIC RISK OF CHEMICALS TO HUMANS

PREAMBLE

BACKGROUND

In 1971, the International Agency for Research on Cancer (IARC) initiated a programme on the evaluation of the carcinogenic risk of chemicals to humans with the object of producing monographs on individual chemicals*. The criteria established at that time to evaluate carcinogenic risk to humans were adopted by all the working groups whose deliberations resulted in the first 16 volumes of the *IARC Monograph* series. In October 1977, a joint IARC/WHO *ad hoc* Working Group met to re-evaluate these guiding criteria; this preamble reflects the results of their deliberations(1) and those of a subsequent IARC *ad hoc* Working Group which met in April 1978(2).

OBJECTIVE AND SCOPE

The objective of the programme is to elaborate and publish in the form of monographs critical reviews of data on carcinogenicity for groups of chemicals to which humans are known to be exposed, to evaluate these data in terms of human risk with the help of international working groups of experts in chemical carcinogenesis and related fields, and to indicate where additional research efforts are needed.

The monographs summarize the evidence for the carcinogenicity of individual chemicals and other relevant information. The critical analyses of the data are intended to assist national and international authorities in formulating decisions concerning preventive measures. No recommendations are given concerning legislation, since this depends on risk-benefit evaluations, which seem best made by individual governments and/or international agencies. In this connection, WHO recommendations on food additives(3), drugs(4), pesticides and contaminants(5) and occupational carcinogens(6) are particularly informative.

---

*Since 1972, the programme has undergone considerable expansion, primarily with the scientific collaboration and financial support of the US National Cancer Institute.

The *IARC Monographs* are recognized as an authoritative source of information on the carcinogenicity of environmental chemicals. The first users' survey, made in 1976, indicates that the monographs are consulted routinely by various agencies in 24 countries.

Since the programme began in 1971, 22 volumes have been published(7) in the *IARC Monograph* series, and 456 separate chemical substances have been evaluated (see also cumulative index to the monographs, p. 189). Each volume is printed in 4000 copies and distributed *via* the WHO publications service (see inside covers for a listing of IARC publications and back outside cover for distribution and sales services).

SELECTION OF CHEMICALS FOR MONOGRAPHS

The chemicals (natural and synthetic, including those which occur as mixtures and in manufacturing processes) are selected for evaluation on the basis of two main criteria: (a) there is evidence of human exposure, and (b) there is some experimental evidence of carcinogenicity and/or there is some evidence or suspicion of a risk to humans. In certain instances, chemical analogues were also considered.

Inclusion of a chemical in a volume does not imply that it is carcinogenic, only that the published data have been examined. The evaluations must be consulted to ascertain the conclusions of the Working Group. Equally, the fact that a chemical has not appeared in a monograph does not mean that it is without carcinogenic hazard.

The scientific literature is surveyed for published data relevant to the monograph programme. In addition, the IARC *Survey of Chemicals Being Tested for Carcinogenicity*(8) often indicates those chemicals that are to be scheduled for future meetings. The major aims of the survey are to prevent unnecessary duplication of research, to increase communication among scientists, and to make a census of chemicals that are being tested and of available research facilities.

As new data on chemicals for which monographs have already been prepared and new principles for evaluating carcinogenic risk receive acceptance, re-evaluations will be made at subsequent meetings, and revised monographs will be published as necessary.

WORKING PROCEDURES

Approximately one year in advance of a meeting of a working group, a list of the substances to be considered is prepared by IARC staff in consultation with other experts. Subsequently, all relevant biological data are collected by IARC; in addition to the published literature, US Public Health Service Publication No. 149(9) has been particularly valuable and has been used in conjunction with other recognized sources of information on chemical carcinogenesis and systems such as CANCERLINE, MEDLINE and TOX LINE. The major collection of data and the preparation of first drafts for the sections on chemical and physical properties, on production, use, occurrence and on analysis are carried out by SRI International under a separate contract with the US National Cancer Institute. Most of the data so obtained on production, use and occurrence refer to the United States and Japan; SRI International and IARC supplement this information with that from other sources in Europe. Bibliographical sources for data on mutagenicity and teratogenicity are the Environmental Mutagen Information Center and the Environmental Teratology Information Center, both located at the Oak Ridge National Laboratory, USA.

Six to nine months before the meeting, reprints of articles containing relevant biological data are sent to an expert(s), or are used by the IARC staff, for the preparation of first drafts of the monographs. These drafts are edited by IARC staff and are sent prior to the meeting to all participants of the Working Group for their comments. The Working Group then meets in Lyon for seven to eight days to discuss and finalize the texts of the monographs and to formulate the evaluations. After the meeting, the master copy of each monograph is verified by consulting the original literature, then edited and prepared for reproduction. The monographs are usually published within six months after the Working Group meeting.

DATA FOR EVALUATIONS

With regard to biological data, only reports that have been published or accepted for publication are reviewed by the working groups, although a few exceptions have been made. The monographs do not cite all of the literature on a particular chemical: only those data considered by the Working Group to be relevant to the evaluation of the carcinogenic risk of the chemical to humans are included.

Anyone who is aware of data that have been published or are in press which are relevant to the evaluations of the carcinogenic risk to humans of chemicals for which monographs have appeared is urged to make them available to the Division of Chemical and Biological Carcinogenesis, International Agency for Research on Cancer, Lyon, France.

THE WORKING GROUP

The tasks of the Working Group are five-fold: (a) to ascertain that all data have been collected; (b) to select the data relevant for the evaluation; (c) to ensure that the summaries of the data enable the reader to follow the reasoning of the committee; (d) to judge the significance of the results of experimental and epidemiological studies; and (e) to make an evaluation of the carcinogenic risk of the chemical.

Working Group participants who contributed to the consideration and evaluation of chemicals within a particular volume are listed, with their addresses, at the beginning of each publication (see p. 5). Each member serves as an individual scientist and not as a representative of any organization or government. In addition, observers are often invited from national and international agencies, organizations and industries.

GENERAL PRINCIPLES FOR EVALUATING THE CARCINOGENIC RISK OF CHEMICALS

The widely accepted meaning of the term 'chemical carcinogenesis', and that used in these monographs, is the induction by chemicals of neoplasms that are not usually observed, the earlier induction by chemicals of neoplasms that are usually observed, and/or the induction by chemicals of more neoplasms than are usually found - although fundamentally different mechanisms may be involved in these three situations. Etymologically, the term 'carcinogenesis' means the induction of cancer, that is, of malignant neoplasms; however, the commonly accepted meaning is the induction of various types of neoplasms or of a combination of malignant and benign tumours. In the monographs, the words 'tumour' and 'neoplasm' are used interchangeably (In scientific literature the terms 'tumourigen', 'oncogen', and 'blastomogen', have all been used synonymously with 'carcinogen', although occasionally 'tumourigen' has been used specifically to denote the induction of benign tumours).

Experimental Evidence

Qualitative aspects

Both the interpretation and evaluation of a particular study as well as the overall assessment of the carcinogenic activity of a chemical involve several qualitatively important considerations, including: (a) the experimental parameters under which the chemical was tested, including route of administration and exposure, species, strain, sex, age, etc.; (b) the consistency with which the chemical has been shown to be carcinogenic, e.g., in how many species and at which target organ(s); (c) the spectrum of neoplastic response, from benign neoplasia to multiple malignant tumours; (d) the stage of tumour formation in which a chemical may be involved: some chemicals act as complete carcinogens and have initiating and promoting activity, while others are promoters only; and (e) the possible role of modifying factors.

There are problems not only of differential survival but of differential toxicity, which may be manifested by unequal growth and weight gain in treated and control animals. These complexities should also be considered in the interpretation of data, or, better, in the experimental design.

Many chemicals induce both benign and malignant tumours; few instances are recorded in which only benign neoplasms are induced by chemicals that have been studied extensively. Benign tumours may represent a stage in the evolution of a malignant neoplasm or they may be 'end-points' that do not readily undergo transition to malignancy. If a substance is found to induce only benign tumours in experimental animals, the chemical should be suspected of being a carcinogen and requires further investigation.

Hormonal carcinogenesis

Hormonal carcinogenesis presents certain distinctive features: the chemicals involved occur both endogenously and exogenously; in many instances, long exposure is required; tumours occur in the target tissue in association with a stimulation of non-neoplastic growth, but in some cases, hormones promote the proliferation of tumour cells in a target organ. Hormones that occur in excessive amounts, hormone-mimetic agents and agents that cause hyperactivity or imbalance in the endocrine system may require evaluative methods comparable with those used to identify chemical carcinogens; particular emphasis must be laid on quantitative aspects and duration of exposure. Some chemical carcinogens have significant side effects on the endocrine system, which may also result in hormonal carcinogenesis. Synthetic hormones and anti-hormones can be expected to possess other pharmacological and toxicological actions in addition to those on the endocrine system, and in this respect they must be treated like any other chemical with regard to intrinsic carcinogenic potential.

Quantitative aspects

Dose-response studies are important in the evaluation of carcinogenesis: the confidence with which a carcinogenic effect can be established is strengthened by the observation of an increasing incidence of neoplasms with increasing exposure.

The assessment of carcinogenicity in animals is frequently complicated by recognized differences among the test animals (species, strain, sex, age), route(s) of administration and in dose/duration of exposure; often, target organs at which a cancer occurs and its histological type may vary with these parameters. Nevertheless, indices of carcinogenic potency in particular experimental systems (for instance, the dose-rate required under continuous exposure to halve the probability of the animals remaining tumourless[10]) have been formulated in the hope that, at least among categories of fairly similar agents, such indices may be of some predictive value in other systems, including humans.

Chemical carcinogens differ widely in the dose required to produce a given level of tumour induction, although many of them share common biological properties which include metabolism to reactive (electrophilic[11-13]) intermediates capable of interacting with DNA. The reason for this variation in dose-response is not understood but may be due either to differences within a common metabolic process or to the operation of qualitatively distinct mechanisms.

Statistical analysis of animal studies

Tumours which would have arisen had an animal lived longer may not be observed because of the death of the animal from unrelated causes, and this possibility must be allowed for. Various analytical techniques have been developed which use the assumption of independence of competing risks to allow for the effects of intercurrent mortality on the final numbers of tumour-bearing animals in particular treatment groups.

For externally visible tumours and for neoplasms that cause death, methods such as Kaplan-Meier (i.e., 'life-table', 'product-limit', or 'actuarial') estimates(10), with associated significance tests(14,15), are recommended.

For internal neoplasms which are discovered 'incidentally'(14) at autopsy but which did not cause the death of the host, different estimates(16) and significance tests(14,15) may be necessary for the unbiased study of the numbers of tumour-bearing animals.

All of these methods(10,14-16) can be used to analyse the numbers of animals bearing particular tumour types, but they do not distinguish between animals with one or many such tumours. In experiments which end at a particular fixed time, with the simultaneous sacrifice of many animals, analysis of the total numbers of internal neoplasms per animal found at autopsy at the end of the experiment is straightforward. However, there are no adequate statistical methods for analysing the numbers of particular neoplasms that kill an animal.

Evidence of Carcinogenicity in Humans

Evidence of carcinogenicity in humans can be derived from three types of study, the first two of which usually provide only suggestive evidence: (1) reports concerning individual cancer patients (case reports), including a history of exposure to the supposed carcinogenic agent; (2) descriptive epidemiological studies in which the incidence of cancer in human populations is found to vary (spatially or temporally) with exposure to the agent; and (3) analytical epidemiological studies (e.g., case-control or cohort studies) in which individual exposure to the agent is found to be associated with an increased risk of cancer.

An analytical study that shows a positive association between an agent and a cancer may be interpreted as implying causality to a greater or lesser extent, if the following criteria are met: (a) there is no identifiable positive bias (By 'positive bias' is meant the operation of factors in study design or execution which lead erroneously to a more strongly positive association between an agent and disease than in fact exists. Examples of positive bias include, in case-control studies, better documentation of exposure to the agent for cases than for controls, and, in cohort studies, the use of better means of detecting cancer in individuals exposed to the agent than in individuals not exposed); (b) the possibility of positive confounding has been considered (By 'positive confounding' is meant a situation in which the relationship between an agent and a disease is rendered more strongly positive than it truly is as a result of an association between that agent and another agent which either causes or prevents the disease. An example of positive confounding is the association between coffee consumption and lung cancer, which results from their joint association with cigarette smoking); (c) the association is unlikely to be due to chance alone; (d) the association is strong; and (e) there is a dose-response relationship.

In some instances, a single epidemiological study may be strongly indicative of a cause-effect relationship; however, the most convincing evidence of causality comes when several independent studies done under different circumstances result in 'positive' findings.

Analytical epidemiological studies that show no association between an agent and a cancer ('negative' studies) should be interpreted according to criteria analogous to those listed above: (a) there is no identifiable negative bias; (b) the possibility of negative confounding has been considered; and (c) the possible effects of misclassification of exposure or outcome have been weighed.

In addition, it must be recognized that in any study there are confidence limits around the estimate of association or relative risk. In a study regarded as 'negative', the upper confidence limit may indicate a relative risk substantially greater than unity; in that case, the study excludes only relative risks that are above this upper limit. This usually means that a 'negative' study must be large to be convincing. Confidence in a 'negative' result is increased when several independent studies carried out under different circumstances are in agreement.

Finally, a 'negative' study may be considered to be relevant only to dose levels within or below the range of those observed in the study and is pertinent only if sufficient time has elapsed since first human exposure to the agent. Experience with human cancers of known etiology suggests that the period from first exposure to a chemical carcinogen to development of clinically observed cancer is usually measured in decades and may be in excess of 30 years.

Experimental Data Relevant to the Evaluation of Carcinogenic Risk to Humans

No adequate criteria are presently available to interpret experimental carcinogenicity data directly in terms of carcinogenic potential for humans. Nonetheless, utilizing data collected from appropriate tests in animals, positive extrapolations to possible human risk can be approximated.

Information compiled from the first 17 volumes of the *IARC Monographs*(17-19) shows that of about 26 chemicals or manufacturing processes now generally accepted to cause cancer in humans, all but possibly two (arsenic and benzene) of those which have been tested appropriately produce cancer in at least one animal species. For several (aflatoxins, 4-aminobiphenyl, diethylstilboestrol, melphalan, mustard gas and vinyl chloride), evidence of carcinogenicity in experimental animals preceded evidence obtained from epidemiological studies or case reports.

In general, the evidence that a chemical produces tumours in experimental animals is of two degrees: (a) *sufficient evidence* of carcinogenicity is provided by the production of malignant tumours; and (b) *limited evidence* of carcinogenicity reflects qualitative and/or quantitative limitations of the experimental results.

For many of the chemicals evaluated in the first 20 volumes of the *IARC Monographs* for which there is *sufficient evidence* of carcinogenicity in animals, data relating to carcinogenicity for humans are either insufficient or nonexistent. In the absence of adequate data on humans, it is reasonable, for practical purposes, to regard such chemicals as if they presented a carcinogenic risk to humans.

Sufficient evidence of carcinogenicity is provided by experimental studies that show an increased incidence of malignant tumours: (i) in multiple species or strains, and/or (ii) in multiple experiments (routes and/or doses), and/or (iii) to an unusual degree (with regard to incidence, site, type and/or precocity of onset). Additional evidence may be provided by data concerning dose-response, mutagenicity or structure.

In the present state of knowledge, it would be difficult to define a predictable relationship between the dose (mg/kg bw/day) of a particular chemical required to produce cancer in test animals and the dose which would produce a similar incidence of cancer in humans. The available data suggest, however, that such a relationship may exist(20,21), at least for certain classes of carcinogenic chemicals. Data that provide *sufficient evidence* of carcinogenicity in test animals may therefore be used in an approximate quantitative evaluation of the human risk at some given exposure level, provided that the nature of the chemical concerned and the physiological, pharmacological and toxicological differences between the test animals and humans are taken into account. However, no acceptable methods are currently available for quantifying the possible errors in such a procedure, whether it is used to generalize between species or to extrapolate from high to low doses. The methodology for such quantitative extrapolation to humans requires further development.

Evidence for the carcinogenicity of some chemicals in experimental animals may be limited for two reasons. Firstly, experimental data may be restricted to such a point that it is not possible to determine a causal relationship between administration of a chemical and the development of a particular lesion in the animals. Secondly, there are certain neoplasms, including lung tumours and hepatomas in mice, which have been considered of lesser significance than neoplasms occurring at other sites for the purpose of evaluating the carcinogenicity of chemicals. Such tumours occur spontaneously in high incidence in these animals, and their malignancy is often difficult to establish. An evaluation of the significance of these tumours following administration of a chemical is the responsibility of particular Working Groups preparing individual monographs, and it has not been possible to set down rigid guidelines; the relevance of these tumours must be determined by considerations which include experimental design and completeness of reporting.

Some chemicals for which there is *limited evidence* of carcinogenicity in animals have also been studied in humans with, in general, inconclusive results. While such chemicals may indeed be carcinogenic to humans, more experimental and epidemiological investigation is required.

Hence *'sufficient evidence'* of carcinogenicity and *'limited evidence'* of carcinogenicity do not indicate categories of chemicals: the inherent definitions of those terms indicate varying degrees of experimental evidence, which may change if and when new data on the chemicals become available. The main drawback to any rigid classification of chemicals with regard to their carcinogenic capacity is the as yet incomplete knowledge of the mechanism(s) of carcinogenesis.

In recent years, several short-term tests for the detection of potential carcinogens have been developed. When only inadequate experimental data are available, positive results in validated short-term tests (see p. 23) are an indication that the compound is a potential carcinogen and that it should be tested in animals for an assessment of its carcinogenicity. Negative results from short-term tests cannot be considered sufficient evidence to rule out carcinogenicity. Whether short-term tests will eventually be as reliable as long-term tests in predicting carcinogenicity in humans will depend on further demonstrations of consistency with long-term experiments and with data from humans.

EXPLANATORY NOTES ON THE MONOGRAPH CONTENTS

Chemical and Physical Data (Section 1)

The Chemical Abstracts Service Registry Number and the latest Chemical Abstracts Primary Name (9th Collective Index)(22) are recorded in section 1. Other synonyms and trade names are given, but no comprehensive list is provided. Further, some of the trade names are those of mixtures in which the compound being evaluated is only one of the ingredients.

The structural and molecular formulae, molecular weight and chemical and physical properties are given. The properties listed refer to the pure substance, unless otherwise specified, and include, in particular, data that might be relevant to carcinogenicity (e.g., lipid solubility) and those that concern identification. A separate description of the composition of technical products includes available information on impurities and formulated products.

Production, Use, Occurrence and Analysis (Section 2)

The purpose of section 2 is to provide indications of the extent of past and present human exposure to the chemical.

Synthesis

Since cancer is a delayed toxic effect, the dates of first synthesis and of first commercial production of the chemical are provided. In addition, methods of synthesis used in past and present commercial production are described. This information allows a reasonable estimate to be made of the date before which no human exposure could have occurred.

Production

Since Europe, Japan and the United States are reasonably representative industrialized areas of the world, most data on production, foreign trade and uses are obtained from those countries. It should not, however, be inferred that those nations are the sole or even the major sources or users of any individual chemical.

Production and foreign trade data are obtained from both governmental and trade publications by chemical economists in the three geographical areas. In some cases, separate production data on organic chemicals manufactured in the United States are not available because their publication could disclose confidential information. In such cases, an indication of the minimum quantity produced can be inferred from the number of companies reporting commercial production. Each company is required to report on individual chemicals if the sales value or the weight of the annual production exceeds a specified minimum level. These levels vary for chemicals classified for different uses, e.g., medicinals and plastics; in fact, the minimal annual sales value is between $1000 and $50,000 and the minimal annual weight of production is between 450 and 22,700 kg. Data on production in some European countries are obtained by means of general questionnaires sent to companies thought to produce the compounds being evaluated. Information from the completed questionnaires is compiled by country, and the resulting estimates of production are included in the individual monographs.

Use

Information on uses is meant to serve as a guide only and is not complete. It is usually obtained from published data but is often complemented by direct contact with manufacturers of the chemical. In the case of drugs, mention of their therapeutic uses does not necessarily represent current practice nor does it imply judgement as to their clinical efficacy.

Statements concerning regulations and standards (e.g., pesticide registrations, maximum levels permitted in foods, occupational standards and allowable limits) in specific countries are mentioned as examples only. They may not reflect the most recent situation, since such legislation is in a constant state of change; nor should it be taken to imply that other countries do not have similar regulations.

Occurrence

Information on the occurrence of a chemical in the environment is obtained from published data including that derived from the monitoring and surveillance of levels of the chemical in occupational environments, air, water, soil, foods and tissues of animals and humans. When available, data on the generation, persistence and bioaccumulation of a chemical are also included.

Analysis

The purpose of the section on analysis is to give the reader an indication, rather than a complete review, of methods cited in the literature. No attempt is made to evaluate critically or to recommend any of the methods.

Biological Data Relevant to the Evaluation of Carcinogenic Risk to Humans (Section 3)

In general, the data recorded in section 3 are summarized as given by the author; however, comments made by the Working Group on certain shortcomings of reporting, of statistical analysis or of experimental design are given in square brackets. The nature and extent of impurities/contaminants in the chemicals being tested are given when available.

Carcinogenicity studies in animals

The monographs are not intended to cover all reported studies. Some studies are purposely omitted (a) because they are inadequate, as judged from previously described criteria(23-26) (e.g., too short a duration, too few animals, poor survival); (b) because they only confirm findings that have already been fully described; or (c) because they are judged irrelevant for the purpose of the evaluation. In certain cases, however, such studies are mentioned briefly, particularly when the information is considered to be a useful supplement to other reports or when it is the only data available. Their inclusion does not, however, imply acceptance of the adequacy of their experimental design and/or of the analysis and interpretation of their results.

Mention is made of all routes of administration by which the compound has been adequately tested and of all species in which relevant tests have been done(5,26). In most cases, animal strains are given (General characteristics of mouse strains have been reviewed (27)). Quantitative data are given to indicate the order of magnitude of the effective carcinogenic doses. In general, the doses and schedules are indicated as they appear in the original paper; sometimes units have been converted for easier comparison. Experiments on the carcinogenicity of known metabolites, chemical precursors, analogues and derivatives, and experiments on factors that modify the carcinogenic effect are also reported.

Other relevant biological data

Lethality data are given when available, and other data on toxicity are included when considered relevant. The metabolic data are restricted to studies that show the metabolic fate of the chemical in animals and humans, and comparisons of data from animals and humans are made when possible. Information is also given on absorption, distribution, excretion and placental transfer.

Embryotoxicity and teratogenicity

Data on teratogenicity from studies in experimental animals and from observations in humans are also included. There appears to be no causal relationship between teratogenicity (28) and carcinogenicity, but chemicals often have both properties. Evidence of teratogenicity suggests transplacental transfer, which is a prerequisite for transplacental carcinogenesis.

Indirect tests (mutagenicity and other short-term tests)

Data from indirect tests are also included. Since most of these tests have the advantage of taking less time and being less expensive than mammalian carcinogenicity studies, they are generally known as 'short-term' tests. They comprise assay procedures which rely on the induction of biological and biochemical effects in *in vivo* and/or *in vitro* systems. The endpoint of the majority of these tests is the production not of neoplasms in animals but of changes at the molecular, cellular or multicellular level: these include the induction of DNA damage and repair, mutagenesis in bacteria and other organisms, transformation of mammalian cells in culture, and other systems.

The short-term tests are proposed for use (a) in predicting potential carcinogenicity in the absence of carcinogenicity data in animals, (b) as a contribution in deciding which chemicals should be tested in animals, (c) in identifying active fractions of complex mixtures containing carcinogens, (d) for recognizing active metabolites of known carcinogens in human and/or animal body fluids and (e) to help elucidate mechanisms of carcinogenesis.

Although the theory that cancer is induced as a result of somatic mutation suggests that agents which damage DNA *in vivo* may be carcinogens, the precise relevance of short-term tests to the mechanism by which cancer is induced is not known. Predictions of potential carcinogenicity are currently based on correlations between responses in short-term tests and data from animal carcinogenicity and/or human epidemiological studies. This approach is limited because the number of chemicals known to be carcinogenic in humans is insufficient to provide a basis for validation, and most validation studies involve chemicals that have been evaluated for carcinogenicity only in animals. The selection of chemicals is in turn limited to those classes for which data on carcinogenicity are available. The results of validation studies could be strongly influenced by such selection of chemicals and by the proportion of carcinogens in the series of chemicals tested; this should be kept in mind when evaluating the predictivity of a particular test. The usefulness of any test is reflected by its ability to classify carcinogens and noncarcinogens, using the animal data as a standard; however, animal tests may not always provide a perfect standard. The attainable level of correlation between short-term tests and animal bioassays is still under investigation.

Since many chemicals require metabolism to an active form, tests that do not take this into account may fail to detect certain potential carcinogens. The metabolic activation systems used in short-term tests (e.g., the cell-free systems used in bacterial tests) are meant to approximate the metabolic capacity of the whole organism. Each test has its advantages and limitations; thus, more confidence can be placed in the conclusions when negative or positive results for a chemical are confirmed in several such test systems. Deficiencies in metabolic competence may lead to misclassification of chemicals, which means that not all tests are suitable for assessing the potential carcinogenicity of all classes of compounds.

The present state of knowledge does not permit the selection of a specific test(s) as the most appropriate for identifying potential carcinogenicity. Before the results of a particular test can be considered to be fully acceptable for predicting potential carcinogenicity, certain criteria should be met: (a) the test should have been validated with respect to known animal carcinogens and found to have a high capacity for discriminating between carcinogens and noncarcinogens, and (b), when possible, a structurally related carcinogen(s) and noncarcinogen(s) should have been tested simultaneously with the chemical in question. The results should have been reproduced in different laboratories, and a prediction of carcinogenicity should have been confirmed in additional test systems. Confidence in positive results is increased if a mechanism of action can be deduced and if appropriate dose-response data are available. For optimum usefulness, data on purity must be given.

The short-term tests in current use that have been the most extensively validated are the *Salmonella typhimurium* plate-incorporation assay(29-33), the X-linked recessive lethal test in *Drosophila melanogaster*(34), unscheduled DNA synthesis(35) and *in vitro* transformation(33,36). Each is compatible with current concepts of the possible mechanism(s) of carcinogenesis.

An adequate assessment of the genetic activity of a chemical depends on data from a wide range of test systems. The monographs include, therefore, data not only from those already mentioned, but also on the induction of point mutations in other systems(37-42), on structural(43) and numerical chromosome aberrations, including dominant lethal effects (44), on mitotic recombination in fungi(37) and on sister chromatid exchanges(45-46).

The existence of a correlation between quantitative aspects of mutagenic and carcinogenic activity has been suggested (5,44-50). but it is not sufficiently well established to allow general use.

Further information about mutagenicity and other short-term tests is given in references 45-53.

Case reports and epidemiological studies

Observations in humans are summarized in this section.

Summary of Data Reported and Evaluation (Section 4)

Section 4 summarizes the relevant data from animals and humans and gives the critical views of the Working Group on those data.

Experimental data

Data relevant to the evaluation of the carcinogenicity of a chemical in animals are summarized in this section. Results from validated mutagenicity and other short-term tests are reported if the Working Group considered the data to be relevant. Dose-response data are given when available. An assessment of the carcinogenicity of the chemical in animals is made on the basis of all of the available data.

The animal species mentioned are those in which the carcinogenicity of the substance was clearly demonstrated. The route of administration used in experimental animals that is similar to the possible human exposure is given particular mention. Tumour sites are also indicated. If the substance has produced tumours after prenatal exposure or in single-dose experiments, this is indicated.

Human data

Case reports and epidemiological studies that are considered to be pertinent to an assessment of human carcinogenicity are described. Human exposure to the chemical is summarized on the basis of data on production, use and occurrence. Other biological data which are considered to be relevant are also mentioned. An assessment of the carcinogenicity of the chemical in humans is made on the basis of all of the available evidence.

Evaluation

This section comprises the overall evaluation by the Working Group of the carcinogenic risk of the chemical to humans. All of the data in the monograph, and particularly the summarized information on experimental and human data, are considered in order to make this evaluation.

References

1. IARC (1977) IARC Monograph Programme on the Evaluation of the Carcinogenic Risk of Chemicals to Humans. Preamble. *IARC intern. tech. Rep. No. 77/002*

2. IARC (1978) Chemicals with *sufficient evidence* of carcinogenicity in experimental animals - *IARC Monographs* volumes 1-17. *IARC intern. tech. Rep. No. 78/003*

3. WHO (1961) Fifth Report of the Joint FAO/WHO Expert Committee on Food Additives. Evaluation of carcinogenic hazard of food additives. *WHO tech. Rep. Ser., No. 220*, pp. 5, 18, 19

4. WHO (1969) Report of a WHO Scientific Group. Principles for the testing and evaluation of drugs for carcinogenicity. *WHO tech. Rep. Ser., No. 426*, pp. 19, 21, 22

5. WHO (1974) Report of a WHO Scientific Group. Assessment of the carcinogenicity and mutagenicity of chemicals. *WHO tech. Rep. Ser., No. 546*

6. WHO (1964) Report of a WHO Expert Committee. Prevention of cancer. *WHO tech. Rep. Ser., No. 276*, pp. 29, 30

7. IARC (1972-1978) *IARC Monographs on the Evaluation of the Carcinogenic Risk of Chemicals to Humans*, Volumes 1-18, Lyon, France

    Volume 1 (1972) Some Inorganic Substances, Chlorinated Hydrocarbons, Aromatic Amines, *N*-Nitroso Compounds and Natural Products (19 monographs), 184 pages

    Volume 2 (1973) Some Inorganic and Organometallic Compounds (7 monographs), 181 pages

    Volume 3 (1973) Certain Polycyclic Aromatic Hydrocarbons and Heterocyclic Compounds (17 monographs), 271 pages

    Volume 4 (1974) Some Aromatic Amines, Hydrazine and Related Substances, *N*-Nitroso Compounds and Miscellaneous Alkylating Agents (28 monographs), 286 pages

    Volume 5 (1974) Some Organochlorine Pesticides (12 monographs), 241 pages

    Volume 6 (1974) Sex Hormones (15 monographs), 243 pages

Volume 7 (1974) Some Anti-thyroid and Related Substances, Nitrofurans and Industrial Chemicals (23 monographs), 326 pages

Volume 8 (1975) Some Aromatic Azo Compounds (32 monographs), 357 pages

Volume 9 (1975) Some Aziridines, *N-, S-* and *O*-Mustards and Selenium (24 monographs), 268 pages

Volume 10 (1976) Some Naturally Occurring Substances (32 monographs), 353 pages

Volume 11 (1976) Cadmium, Nickel, Some Epoxides, Miscellaneous Industrial Chemicals and General Considerations on Volatile Anaesthetics (24 monographs), 306 pages

Volume 12 (1976) Some Carbamates, Thiocarbamates and Carbazides (24 monographs), 282 pages

Volume 13 (1977) Some Miscellaneous Pharmaceutical Substances (17 monographs), 255 pages

Volume 14 (1977) Asbestos (1 monograph), 106 pages

Volume 15 (1977) Some Fumigants, the Herbicides 2,4-D and 2,4,5-T, Chlorinated Dibenzodioxins and Miscellaneous Industrial Chemicals (18 monographs), 354 pages

Volume 16 (1978) Some Aromatic Amines and Related Nitro Compounds - Hair Dyes, Colouring Agents, and Miscellaneous Industrial Chemicals (32 monographs), 400 pages

Volume 17 (1978) Some *N*-Nitroso Compounds (17 monographs), 365 pages

Volume 18 (1978) Polychlorinated Biphenyls and Polybrominated Biphenyls (2 monographs), 140 pages

Volume 19 (1979) Some Monomers, Plastics and Synthetic Elastomers, and Acrolein (17 monographs), 513 pages

Volume 20 (1979) Some Halogenated Hydrocarbons (25 monographs), 609 pages

Volume 21 (1979) Sex Hormones (II) (22 monographs), 583 pages

Volume 22 (1980) Some Non-Nutritive Sweetening Agents (2 monographs), 208 pages

8.   IARC (1973-1979) *Information Bulletin on the Survey of Chemicals Being Tested for Carcinogenicity*, Numbers 1-8, Lyon, France

      Number 1 (1973) 52 pages
      Number 2 (1973) 77 pages
      Number 3 (1974) 67 pages
      Number 4 (1974) 97 pages
      Number 5 (1975) 88 pages
      Number 6 (1976) 360 pages
      Number 7 (1978) 460 pages
      Number 8 (1979) 604 pages

9.   PHS 149 (1951-1976) Public Health Service Publication No. 149, *Survey of Compounds which have been Tested for Carcinogenic Activity*, Washington DC, US Government Printing Office

      1951   Hartwell, J.L., 2nd ed., Literature up to 1947 on 1329 compounds, 583 pages

      1957   Shubik, P. & Hartwell, J.L., Supplement 1, Literature for the years 1948-1953 on 981 compounds, 388 pages

      1969   Shubik, P. & Hartwell, J.L., edited by Peters, J.A., Supplement 2, Literature for the years 1954-1960 on 1048 compounds, 655 pages

      1971   National Cancer Institute, Literature for the years 1968-1969 on 882 compounds, 653 pages

      1973   National Cancer Institute, Literature for the years 1961-1967 on 1632 compounds, 2343 pages

      1974   National Cancer Institute, Literature for the years 1970-1971 on 750 compounds, 1667 pages

      1976   National Cancer Institute, Literature for the years 1972-1973 on 966 compounds, 1638 pages

10.   Pike, M.C. & Roe, F.J.C. (1963) An actuarial method of analysis of an experiment in two-stage carcinogenesis. *Br. J. Cancer, 17*, 605-610

11.   Miller, E.C. & Miller, J.A. (1966) Mechanisms of chemical carcinogenesis: nature of proximate carcinogens and interactions with macromolecules. *Pharmacol. Rev., 18*, 805-838

12.   Miller, J.A. (1970) Carcinogenesis by chemicals: an overview - G.H.A. Clowes Memorial Lecture. *Cancer Res., 30*, 559-576

13. Miller, J.A. & Miller, E.C. (1976) *The metabolic activation of chemical carcinogens to reactive electrophiles.* In: Yuhas, J.M., Tennant, R.W. & Reagon, J.D., eds, *Biology of Radiation Carcinogenesis,* New York, Raven Press

14. Peto, R. (1974) Guidelines on the analysis of tumours rates and death rates in experimental animals. *Br. J. Cancer, 29,* 101-105

15. Peto, R. (1975) Letter to the editor. *Br. J. Cancer, 31,* 697-699

16. Hoel, D.G. & Walburg, H.E., Jr (1972) Statistical analysis of survival experiments. *J. natl Cancer Inst., 49,* 361-372

17. Tomatis, L. (1977) *The value of long-term testing for the implementation of primary prevention.* In: Hiatt, H.H., Watson, J.D. & Winsten, J.A., eds, *Origins of Human Cancer,* Book C, Cold Spring Harbor, N.Y., Cold Spring Harbor Laboratory, pp. 1339-1357

18. IARC (1977) *Annual Report 1977,* Lyon, International Agency for Research on Cancer, p. 94

19. Tomatis, L., Agthe, C., Bartsch, H., Huff, J., Montesano, R., Saracci, R., Walker, E. & Wilbourn, J. (1978) Evaluation of the carcinogenicity of chemicals: a review of the IARC Monograph Programme, 1971-1977. *Cancer Res., 38,* 877-885

20. Rall, D.P. (1977) *Species differences in carcinogenesis testing.* In: Hiatt, H.H., Watson, J.D. & Winsten, J.A., eds, *Origins of Human Cancer,* Book C, Cold Spring Harbor, N.Y., Cold Spring Harbor Laboratory, pp. 1383-1390

21. National Academy of Sciences (NAS) (1975) *Contemporary Pest Control Practices and Prospects: the Report of the Executive Committee,* Washington DC

22. Chemical Abstracts Service (1978) *Chemical Abstracts Ninth Collective Index (9CI), 1972-1976,* Vols 76-85, Columbus, Ohio

23. WHO (1958) Second Report of the Joint FAO/WHO Expert Committee on Food Additives. Procedures for the testing of intentional food additives to establish their safety for use. *WHO tech. Rep. Ser., No. 144*

24. WHO (1967) Scientific Group. Procedures for investigating intentional and unintentional food additives. *WHO tech. Rep. Ser., No. 348*

25. Berenblum, I., ed (1969) Carcinogenicity testing. *UICC tech. Rep. Ser., 2*

26. Sontag, J.M., Page, N.P. & Saffiotti, U. (1976) Guidelines for carcinogen bioassay in small rodents. *Natl Cancer Inst. Carcinog. tech. Rep. Ser., No. 1*

27. Committee on Standardized Genetic Nomenclature for Mice (1972) Standardized nomenclature for inbred strains of mice. Fifth listing. *Cancer Res., 32*, 1609-1646

28. Wilson, J.G. & Fraser, F.C. (1977) *Handbook of Teratology*, New York, Plenum Press

29. Ames, B.N., Durston, W.E., Yamasaki, E. & Lee, F.D. (1973) Carcinogens are mutagens: a simple test system combining liver homogenates for activation and bacteria for detection. *Proc. natl Acad. Sci. (USA), 70,* 2281-2285

30. McCann, J., Choi, E., Yamasaki, E. & Ames, B.N. (1975) Detection of carcinogens as mutagens in the *Salmonella*/microsome test: assay of 300 chemicals. *Proc. natl Acad. Sci. (USA), 72*, 5135-5139

31. McCann, J. & Ames, B.N. (1976) Detection of carcinogens as mutagens in the *Salmonella*/microsome test: assay of 300 chemicals: discussion. *Proc. natl Acad. Sci. (USA), 73*, 950-954

32. Sugimura, T., Sato, S., Nagao, M., Yahagi, T., Matsushima, T., Seino, Y., Takeuchi, M. & Kawachi, T. (1977) *Overlapping of carcinogens and mutagens.* In: Magee, P.N., Takayama, S., Sugimura, T. & Matsushima, T., eds, *Fundamentals in Cancer Prevention*, Baltimore, University Park Press, pp. 191-215

33. Purchase, I.F.M., Longstaff, E., Ashby, J., Styles, J.A., Anderson, D., Lefevre, P.A. & Westwood, F.R. (1976) Evaluation of six short term tests for detecting organic chemical carcinogens and recommendations for their use. *Nature, 264*, 624-627

34. Vogel, E. & Sobels, F.H. (1976) *The function of* Drosophila *in genetic toxicology testing.* In: Hollaender, A., ed., *Chemical Mutagens: Principles and Methods for Their Detection*, Vol. 4, New York, Plenum Press, pp. 93-142

35. San, R.H.C. & Stich, H.F. (1975) DNA repair synthesis of cultured human cells as a rapid bioassay for chemical carcinogens. *Int. J. Cancer, 16*, 284-291

36. Pienta, R.J., Poiley, J.A. & Lebherz, W.B. (1977) Morphological transformation of early passage golden Syrian hamster embryo cells derived from cryopreserved primary cultures as a reliable *in vitro* bioassay for identifying diverse carcinogens. *Int. J. Cancer, 19*, 642-655

37. Zimmermann, F.K. (1975) Procedures used in the induction of mitotic recombination and mutation in the yeast *Saccharomyces cerevisiae*. *Mutat. Res., 31,* 71-86

38. Ong, T.-M. & de Serres, F.J. (1972) Mutagenicity of chemical carcinogens in *Neurospora crassa*. *Cancer Res., 32,* 1890-1893

39. Huberman, E. & Sachs, L. (1976) Mutability of different genetic loci in mammalian cells by metabolically activated carcinogenic polycyclic hydrocarbons. *Proc. natl Acad. Sci. (USA), 73,* 188-192

40. Krahn, D.F. & Heidelburger, C. (1977) Liver homogenate-mediated mutagenesis in Chinese hamster V79 cells by polycyclic aromatic hydrocarbons and aflatoxins. *Mutat. Res., 46,* 27-44

41. Kuroki, T., Drevon, C. & Montesano, R. (1977) Microsome-mediated mutagenesis in V79 Chinese hamster cells by various nitrosamines. *Cancer Res., 37,* 1044-1050

42. Searle, A.G. (1975) The specific locus test in the mouse. *Mutat. Res., 31,* 277-290

43. Evans, H.J. & O'Riordan, M.L.(1975) Human peripheral blood lymphocytes for the analysis of chromosome aberrations in mutagen tests. *Mutat. Res., 31,* 135-148

44. Epstein, S.S., Arnold, E., Andrea, J., Bass, W. & Bishop, Y. (1972) Detection of chemical mutagens by the dominant lethal assay in the mouse. *Toxicol. appl. Pharmacol., 23,* 288-325

45. Perry, P. & Evans, H.J. (1975) Cytological detection of mutagen-carcinogen exposure by sister chromatid exchanges. *Nature, 258,* 121-125

46. Stetka, D.G. & Wolff, S. (1976) Sister chromatid exchanges as an assay for genetic damage induced by mutagen-carcinogens. I. *In vivo* test for compounds requiring metabolic activation. *Mutat. Res., 41,* 333-342

47. Bartsch, H. & Grover, P.L. (1976) *Chemical carcinogenesis and mutagenesis.* In: Symington, T. & Carter, R.L.,eds, *Scientific Foundations of Oncology*, Vol. IX, *Chemical Carcinogenesis,* London, Heinemann Medical Books Ltd, pp. 334-342

48. Hollaender, A., ed.(1971a,b, 1973, 1976) *Chemical Mutagens: Principles and Methods for Their Detection,* Vols 1-4, New York, Plenum Press

49. Montesano, R. & Tomatis, L., eds (1974) *Chemical Carcinogenesis Essays,* Lyon *(IARC Scientific Publications No. 10)*

50. Ramel, C., ed. (1973) Evaluation of genetic risk of environmental chemicals: report of a symposium held at Skokloster, Sweden, 1972. *Ambio Spec. Rep., No. 3*

51. Stoltz, D.R., Poirier, L.A., Irving, C.C., Stich, H.F., Weisburger, J.H. & Grice, H.C. (1974) Evaluation of short-term tests for carcinogenicity. *Toxicol. appl. Pharmacol., 29,* 157-180

52. Montesano, R., Bartsch, H. & Tomatis, L., eds (1976) *Screening Tests in Chemical Carcinogenesis*, Lyon *(IARC Scientific Publications No. 12)*

53. Committee 17 (1976) Environmental mutagenic hazards. *Science, 187,* 503-514

GENERAL REMARKS ON THE SUBSTANCES CONSIDERED

In this twenty-second volume of the *IARC Monographs* series, certain synthetic non-nutritive sweeteners and their major metabolites or impurities have been evaluated. Thus, the monograph on cyclamates covers not only the free acid and the sodium and calcium salts, but also cyclohexylamine and dicyclohexylamine. Similarly, *ortho*-toluenesulphonamide is included in the monograph on saccharin and its sodium and calcium salts. It should be noted that the term 'saccharin' is sometimes used here generically to include not only the acid form but also the salts.

Saccharin and cyclamates (and often a mixture of both) have been used for many years as artificial sweeteners and as additives to food and drinks in the place of sugar. They are also used in diets for weight reduction and for control of diabetes and in cosmetics and pharmaceutical products; in addition, saccharin has been used for industrial purposes, notably as a brightener in nickel-plating baths.

The impurities of commercial cyclamate and saccharin products evaluated in this volume are also chemicals of a significant commercial importance themselves. Cyclohexylamine is the key intermediate in the commercial synthesis of cyclamates, and *ortho*-toluenesulphonamide has the same function in one of the two commercial processes used to make saccharin. The two cyclohexylamines are used to produce corrosion inhibitors and rubber-processing chemicals, while *ortho*-toluenesulphonamide is a constituent of a plasticizer used to improve the flow properties of a variety of resins.

The Working Group was unimpressed with the relatively large number of experimental studies on cyclamates, saccharin and related compounds, most of which were found to be inadequate for one reason or another. However, due to the widespread general and scientific interest in artificial sweeteners and the serious and far-reaching repercussions on regulatory and public policy decisions, the Working Group decided to include all available published reports and abstracts for analysis and comments. It was not their intent to formulate a new precedent for presentation of data in these monographs, but it was felt necessary to attempt to analyse fully all of the available data.

Analysis of the experimental data on the carcinogenicity of cyclamates, saccharin and related compounds led the Working Group to recommend that detailed examination of all tissues and organs from test animals become part of an acceptable experimental design. Concentration on any one organ, such as the bladder, to the exclusion of other sites that might react to any test substance should be discouraged. These observations highlight the need for acceptable criteria of adequacy of experiments for determining carcinogenicity, expecially for compounds that are of only moderate or low potency. Doses of several grams per kilogram body weight of both saccharin and cyclamates are required to produce toxic effects in chronic and acute toxicity tests in animals.

Despite much public discussion, there is little evidence that artificial sweeteners have embryotoxic or teratogenic effects in mammals. The two reports in the literature that described teratogenic effects of both saccharin and cyclamates were either not confirmed in the same laboratory or the validity of the data has been questioned with respect to experimental design.

Varying amounts of impurities occur in commercial saccharin, depending on the method of synthesis. The structures of many of these impurities have not yet been identified, and many have not been adequately tested for their adverse biological effects. Since in many instances the concentrations of such impurities in test samples were not determined, the equivocal results often obtained in assays for mutagenicity, embryotoxicity and teratogenicity may therefore be related in part to the presence of biologically active impurities in the test compounds.

A provocative feature of the findings with saccharin is the apparent absence of any evidence for its interaction with cellular macromolecules such as DNA and protein, either by itself or after suitable metabolism. In fact, the Working Group noted the absence of any evidence that saccharin is metabolized to a measurable degree in the mammalian tissues examined. The absence of any binding capacity either before or after metabolism places saccharin apart from the majority of known chemical carcinogens, which are either chemically reactive *per se* (e.g., alkylating agents) or become so after suitable metabolic enzymatic conversion to appropriate derivatives (e.g., electrophilic reactants). These differences between saccharin and many other chemical carcinogens are especially noteworthy.

Saccharin is also negative in point mutation tests *in vitro*, although chromosomal effects are induced by both saccharin and cyclamates *in vivo* and *in vitro*. However, no data on the mutagenicity of cyclamates in point mutation assays have been published, and in neither case has experimentation been sufficient to rule out the possibility of very weak mutagenic activity.

Present evidence thus suggests that saccharin may act as a tumour promoter; this is further supported by results of an *in vitro* cell transformation experiment. The data on cyclamates, saccharin and related compounds thus highlight a developing need to consider the possible importance of promotion and promoters in the overall analysis of the causation of human cancer by chemicals.

The Working Group was impressed by the growing realization that some cancers may be caused by multiple factors, each of which plays a different role in initiating or facilitating a particular step or steps in the carcinogenic process. The multistep nature of cancer development - at least in some organs - and the ability of different chemicals to modify different steps necessitate increased emphasis on the identification of such chemicals and their mechanisms of action. Any exclusive emphasis on chemicals that can initiate cancer development, to the neglect of chemicals that can accelerate steps in the subsequent development of cancer, may impede the discovery of compounds in the environment that enhance cancer development that has been initiated by some other means.

Bladder insertion

This technique has been widely utilized with mice. The test chemical is mixed with a suspending chemical, frequently cholesterol, to form a small pellet, which is inserted surgically into the bladder lumen. Control mice are exposed to pellets made from the suspending chemical only. The test chemical is leached from the pellet by the urine at a rate that varies for each test chemical and each suspending chemical. Thus solubilized, the test chemical passes into and through the bladder. The pellets remain in the bladder lumina for 40 to 60 weeks, when the mice are killed and the bladders inspected both grossly and microscopically. A statistical comparison of the incidence of carcinomas in the test animals with that in the control group is used as a basis for assessing the carcinogenicity of the test compound. The validity of this experimental system has been questioned (IARC, 1978); however, of more than 160 chemicals that have been tested by this method, bladder carcinogenicity has been reported for only 56 (35%). Sixteen compounds (other than sodium cyclamate and sodium saccharin) that have shown bladder carcinogenicity by intravesicular insertion have demonstrated bladder carcinogenicity in one or more species, including humans, when administered systemically (Bryan & Yoshida, 1971).

Confounding factors in experimental studies

1.   Bladder parasites

In several studies reviewed in this monograph, the presence of the bladder parasites *Trichosomoides crassicauda* and *Strongyloides capillaria* was reported. Previous, unrelated studies demonstrated an apparent association between the presence of bladder parasites and an increased risk of bladder tumour formation in rats (Chapman, 1969; Clayson, 1974; Munro *et al.*, 1975). Neoplasia of the urinary tract has also been described in nonhuman primates infected artificially with *Schistosoma haematobium* (Kunz *et al.*, 1972).

In studies in which parasites have either not been reported or not looked for, therefore, an increased tumour incidence must be interpreted with caution.

2.   Mineralization

Mineralization in the urinary tract of rodents can take several forms, including the production of free-lying calculi (usually macroscopically visible stones), intra- or subepithelial deposits and/or microcrystalluria. Burek (1978) reported that in ageing rats microcrystals are produced normally in the urinary tract and excreted in the urine. Evidence from unrelated studies indicates that free-lying bladder calculi may be associated with an increased risk of bladder tumour formation in rodents (Chapman *et al.*, 1973; Clayson, 1974). In the studies reviewed in these two monographs, mineralization was observed, but there was no treatment-related increased incidence of calculi. There was no apparent correlation between other types of mineralization and tumour formation.

General considerations on the evaluation of the epidemiological evidence

The preamble to these monographs (pp. 16-17) considers several general issues which arise in the interpretation of epidemiological data. Points relevant to the study of the association between cancer risk and artificial sweetener consumption are considered below. It was noted by the Working Group that all of the studies cited herein concentrated on risk for bladder cancer and that none were available that considered a possible risk of cancer at other sites.

1.   Trends in incidence or mortality rates

Two studies considered by the Working Group related temporal changes in the incidence or mortality rates of bladder cancer in the general population to changes in the pattern of consumption of artificial sweeteners (Armstrong & Doll, 1974; Burbank & Fraumeni, 1970).

Even if these agents were known to be carcinogenic to humans, the effect that changes in consumption patterns might have on subsequent rates of incidence or mortality could not be readily predicted on the basis of existing knowledge. The magnitude of effect, for example, would depend on the unknown dose-response relationship and the distribution of consumption levels within the population. If the heaviest users were among the young, it might take longer for any effect to appear than if consumption were distributed more uniformly throughout the population, because of the long intervals that are often required before a significant increase in cancer can be seen.

Another difficulty is that small effects could be masked either by concurrent changes in exposure of the general population to other known risk factors, such as tobacco smoking or exposure to certain industrial chemicals. Mortality studies have the additional complication that they are affected by changes in survival rates over time.

2.   Studies on diabetics

Subgroups can be identified that have a greater exposure to artificial sweeteners than that of the general population and these can be examined to see if they have an unusually high risk of cancer. One subgroup that has an increased exposure to artificial sweeteners comprises patients with diabetes mellitus; however, none of the reported studies provide data on individual consumption levels, so that dose-response relationships cannot easily be determined. Comparisons with external ('standard') population rates may not be completely valid due to the fact that diabetics are different both metabolically and with respect to their habits.

3.   Case-control studies

Case-contol studies are a rapid and relatively economical method of quantifying the relationship between individual levels of exposure to an agent and the presence or absence of a disease. The method can allow for known confounding factors (i.e., factors associated both with the exposure and the disease which might cause an indirect association between the two). In case-control studies, subjects are ascertained by the presence of the disease rather than by identification of individuals exposed to the agent. Usually only one disease can be studied at a time. All the case-control studies carried out to date have dealt only with bladder cancer, a site suggested by experimental work.

If the effect of artificial sweeteners is to increase risk by no more than 20-30%, it will be difficult to separate these small effects from the effects of confounding factors, which were either unknown or known and inadequately controlled for in the analysis. Case-control studies are also susceptible to errors of bias arising from the possibility that bladder cancer patients may be more likely to remember and report artificial sweetener use than patients with other diseases, due to the widespread publicity recently given to a possible association between artificial sweeteners and cancer. This will be especially important in interpreting any new studies carried out to further test the hypothesis of an association.

References

Armstrong, B. & Doll, R. (1974) Bladder cancer mortality in England and Wales in relation to cigarette smoking and saccharin consumption. *Br. J. prev. Med., 28*, 233-240

Bryan, G.T. & Yoshida, O. (1971)   Artificial sweeteners as urinary bladder carcinogens. *Arch. environ. Health, 23*, 6-12

Burbank, F. & Fraumeni, J.F., Jr (1970) Synthetic sweeteners consumption and bladder cancer trends in the United States. *Nature, 227*, 296-297

Burek, J.D. (1978) *Pathology of Aging Rats*, West Palm Beach, FL, CRC Press, p. 98

Chapman, W.H. (1969) Infection with *Trichosomoides crassicauda* as a factor in the induction of bladder tumors in rats fed 2-acetylaminofluorine. *Invest. Urol., 7*, 154-159

Chapman, W.H., Kircheim, D. & McRoberts, J.W. (1973) Effects of the urine and calculus formation on the incidence of bladder tumors in rats implanted with paraffin wax pellets. *Cancer Res., 33*, 1225-1229

Clayson, D.B. (1974) Bladder carcinogenesis in rats and mice: possibility of artifacts. *J. natl Cancer Inst., 52*, 1685-1689

IARC (1978) *IARC Monographs on the Evaluation of the Carcinogenic Risk of Chemicals to Man, 16, Some Aromatic Amines and Related Nitro Compounds - Hair Dyes, Colouring Agents and Miscellaneous Industrial Chemicals,* Lyon, p. 19

Kunz, R.E., Cheever, A.W. & Myers, B.J. (1972) Proliferative epithelial lesions of the urinary bladder in nonhuman primates infected with *Schistosoma haematobium.* *J. natl Cancer Inst., 48*, 223-245

Munro, I.C., Moodie, C.A., Krewski, D. & Grice, H.C. (1975) A carcinogenicity study of commercial saccharin in the rat. *Toxicol. appl. Pharmacol., 32*, 513-526

APPENDIX[a]

**REGULATORY STATUS OF NON-NUTRITIVE SWEETENERS CONTAINING CYCLAMATE
AND SACCHARIN**

(+, no restriction on sale or distribution; Ch, distribution only by chemists/pharmacists; P, doctor's
prescription required; B, banned; NM, not mentioned in food laws; —, legal status unknown)

Country	Regulatory status for:		
	Tablets, liquids or powders	Additives in foods	Additives in beverages
AFRICA			
Algeria			
Saccharin (S)	Ch	—	B
Cyclamates (C)	P	B	B
Angola			
S	—	—	—
C	Ch/P	—	—
Burundi			
S	Ch	—	+[b]
C	B	B	B
Canary Islands			
S	Ch	+	—
C	P	—	B
Ethiopia			
S	+	—	+
C	B	B	B
Former French Territories			
S	Ch	—	B
C	P	—	B
Former Portuguese Territories			
S	P	+	+
C	P	NM	NM

Country	Tablets, liquids or powders	Additives in foods	Additives in beverages
Former United Kingdom Territories			
S	+	+	+
C	B	NM	NM
Kenya			
S	+	+	+
C	B	B	B
Morocco			
S	+	+	+
C	+	+	+
Mozambique			
S	P	−	−
C	P	−	−
Nigeria			
S	−	−	+[c]
C	−	−	−
Rhodesia			
S	+	B	B
C	+	+	+
Ruanda			
S	+	−	+[b]
C	B	B	B
Sierra Leone			
S	+	+	+
C	+	+	+
South Africa			
S	+	+[d]	+[d]
C	+	+[e]	+[e]
Sudan			
S	Ch	−	−
C	P	B	B
Tunisia			
S	Ch	+[f]	+[f]
C	Ch	B	B

Country	Tablets, liquids or powders	Additives in foods	Additives in beverages
Uganda			
S	+	+	+
C	B	B	B
Zaire			
S	+	−	+^{g}
C	Ch	−	B
Zambia			
S	+	+	−
C	B	B	B
AMERICA			
Antigua			
S	+	+	+
C	+	+	+
Argentina			
S	Ch	+^{h}	+^{i}
C	Ch	+^{j}	+^{k}
Bahamas			
S	+	−	+^{l}
C	−	−	−
Bermuda			
S	−	−	B
C	B	B	B
Bolivia			
S	Ch	−	B
C	Ch	−	B
Brazil			
S	+^{m}	+^{m}	+^{m}
C	+^{m}	+^{m}	B
Canada			
S	+	+^{n}	+^{n}
C	+^{o}	B	B
Chile			
S	Ch	−	−
C	+^{p}	−	−
Colombia			
S	+	−	+^{q}
C	B	B	B

Country	Tablets, liquids or powders	Additives in foods	Additives in beverages
Costa Rica			
S	+	−	+^{r}
C	Ch	B	B
Dominica			
S	+	−	+
C	+	−	+
Ecuador			
S	+	+	+^{s}
C	Ch^t	B	B
El Salvador			
S	+	−	+^{r}
C	B^u	B	B
French Guyana			
S	Ch	−	B
C	Ch	−	B
French Territories in the Caribbean			
S	Ch	−	B
C	Ch	−	B
Guadeloupe			
S	Ch	−	B
C	Ch	−	B
Guatemala			
S	+	−	+^{r}
C	P/Ch	−	B
Guiana			
S	+	−	+
C	B	−	B
Haiti			
S	+	−	+
C	+	−	+
Honduras			
S	+	−	+^{r}
C	Ch	NM	NM
Jamaica			
S	−	−	−
C	B	B	B

Country	Tablets, liquids or powders	Additives in foods	Additives in beverages
Martinique			
S	Ch	—	B
C	P	—	B
Mexico			
S	+	+	+^{v}
C	+	+	—
Monserrat			
S	+	—	+
C	—	—	+
Most smaller Caribbean countries			
S	+	+^{w}	+^{w}
C	—	+^{w}	+^{w}
Nassau			
S	—	—	+
C	—	—	B
Netherlands Antilles			
S	+	—	—
C	B	B	B
Nicaragua			
S	—	—	+^{r}
C	P/Ch	B	B
Panama			
S	+	—	+^{r}
C	B	B	B
Paraguay			
S	+	—	+^{x}
C	—	—	—
Peru			
S	+	—	B
C	B	B	B
Puerto Rico & US Virgin Islands			
S	+	—	+^{l}
C	B	B	B
Surinam			
S	+	+	+
C	+	+	+
Trinidad			
S	—	—	+^{y}
C	—	+	+^{y}

Country	Tablets, liquids or powders	Additives in foods	Additives in beverages
United States			
S	+	+$^{v}_{/}$	+$^{/}$
C	B	B	B
Uruguay			+^{z}
S	—	—	+^{a_1}
C	P	B	
Venezuela			
S	Ch	—	B
C	Ch	B	B
ASIA			
(Middle East)			
Bahrain			
S	+	—	—
C	B	B	B
Cyprus			
S	+	—	+^{b_1}
C	B	B	B
India			
S	+	+	+^{c_1}
C	B	B	B
Iran			
S	+	—	B
C	B	B	B
Iraq			
S	—	—	B
C	B	B	B
Israel			
S	+	+^{d_1}	B
C	+	B	B
Kuwait			
S	+	—	—
C	P^{n}	—	B
Lebanon			
S	Ch	—	—
C	B	B	B
Pakistan			
S	+	—	+^{q}
C	+	—	+^{q}

Country	Tablets, liquids or powders	Additives in foods	Additives in beverages
Saudi Arabia			
S	+	−	−
C	B	B	B
Sri Lanka			
S	+	−	+[e1]
C	B	−	B
Turkey			
S	+	+	+[d1]
C	B	B	B[d1]
(Far East)			
Cambodia			
S	−	−	B
C	−	B	B
Hong Kong			
S	+	+	I
C	B	B	B
Indonesia			
S	+	+[f1]	+[g1]
C	−	−	+
Japan			
S	−	+[f1]	+[h1]
C	B	B	B
Korea			
S	+	−	+[i1]
C	−	−	−
Malaysia			
S	Ch	B	+[i1]
C	Ch	B	B
Philippines			
S	+	−	+
C	B	B	B
Singapore			
S	+	−	+[i1]
C	B	B	B
South Vietnam			
S	−	−	B
C	−	−	B

Country	Tablets, liquids or powders	Additives in foods	Additives in beverages
Taiwan			
S	−	−	B
C	−	−	B
Thailand			
S	+	−	−
C	Ch/P	−	B
AUSTRALIA AND PACIFIC ISLANDS			
American Samoa, Guam and other US Trust Territories			
S	−	−	$+^{k1}$
C	B	B	B
Australia			
S	+	−	$+^{l1}$
C	Ch	$+^{m1}$	$+^{n1}$
Fiji			
S	−	−	B
C	−	−	B
New Zealand			
S	−	$+^{o1}$	$+^{p1}$
C	+	+	+
EUROPE			
Austria			
S	$+^{n}$	$+^{n}$	$+^{n}$
C	$+^{q1}$	B	B
Belgium			
S	$+^{n}$	$+^{r1}$	$+^{r1}$
C	Ch^{n}	B	B
Bulgaria			
S	−	−	−
C	−	−	B
Czechoslovakia			
S	−	−	+
C	−	−	B
Denmark			
S	$+^{n}$	$+^{s1}$	$+^{t1}$
C	$+^{u1}$	B	B

Country	Tablets, liquids or powders	Additives in foods	Additives in beverages
Federal Republic of Germany			
S	$+^{v1}$	$+^{w1}$	$+^{x1}$
C	$+^{v11}$	$+^{w1}$	$+^{y1}$
Finland			
S	$+$	$+^{z1}$	$+^{n}$
C	$+^{n}$	$+^{z1}$	$+^{a2}$
France			
S	Ch^{n}	$+^{x1}$	$+^{x1}$
C	Ch^{b2}	B	B
German Democratic Republic			
S	$-$	$-$	$-$
C	$-$	$-$	B
Greece			
S	$-$	$-$	$+^{c2}$
C	B	B	B
Hungary			
S	$-$	$-$	$-$
C	$-$	$-$	B
Iceland			
S	$+$	$+$	$+^{d2}$
C	$+$	$+$	$+^{d2}$
Ireland (Republic)			
S	$+^{n}$	$-^{n}$	$+^{n}$
C	$+^{n}$	$+^{n}$	$+^{n}$
Italy			
S	$-^{i1}$	$-^{i1}$	$+^{e2}$
C	$+^{i1}$	$+^{i1}$	$+^{i1'}$
Malta			
S	$+$	$+$	$+$
C	B	B	B
Netherlands			
S	$+^{n}$	$+^{n}$	$+^{n}$
C	Ch^{n}	B	B
Norway			
S	$+^{g2}$	$+^{n}$	$+^{f2}$
C	$+^{g2}$	$+^{g2}$	$+^{g2}$

Country	Tablets, liquids or powders	Additives in foods	Additives in beverages
Poland			
S	—	—	—
C	—	—	B
Portugal			
S	P	+	+^{h2}
C	P/Ch	B	B
Spain			
S	Ch	+	+^{i2}
C	Ch/P	—	+^{i2}
Sweden			
S	+	+^{j2}	+^{j2}
C	B	B	B
Switzerland			
S	+^{n}	+^{k2}	+^{n}
C	+	+	+^{k2}
United Kingdom			
S	+^{n}	+^{l2}	+^{l2}
C	B	B	B
Yugoslavia			
S	—	—	+
C	—	B	B

[a] from Hermes Sweeteners Ltd (1979)

[b] maximum, 75 mg/l; declaration mandatory

[c] maximum, 70 mg/l

[d] maximum, 150 ppm; special labelling mandatory

[e] maximum, 1500 ppm; special labelling mandatory

[f] legal regulation to be followed

[g] maximum, 75 ppm; declaration mandatory

[h] maximum intake, 5 mg/kg bw; special labelling mandatory

[i] maximum, 500 g/l; special labelling mandatory

[j] maximum intake, 50 mg/kg bw; special labelling mandatory

[k] maximum, 2 g/l; special labelling mandatory

l maximum, 406 mg/l; declaration mandatory

m all products under the authority of the Ministry of Health; special labelling mandatory; maximum daily consumption to be stated and 'used under medical advice' (maximum intake: saccharin, 15 mg/kg bw per day; cyclamate, 3.5 g/day per person)

n special labelling mandatory

o advertising not allowed

p not being sold presently

q only in dietetic products; declaration mandatory

r only in dietetic products; maximum, 500 ppm

s declaration mandatory; may be used up to international limits

t advertising not allowed; special labelling mandatory

u allowed only in pharmaceuticals

v declaration mandatory

w imported food products many contain any ingredients permitted in country of origin

x only in dietetic products; authorization of Ministry of Health required

y government approval required prior to use

z only in dietetic products; authorization of Ministry of Health required; maximum, 1500 ppm; special labelling mandatory

a_1 only in dietetic products; authorization of Ministry of Health required; maximum, 20,000 ppm; special labelling mandatory

b_1 only in dietetic products; government approval necessary prior to use

c_1 declaration mandatory; maximum, 100 ppm

d_1 only in dietetic products

e_1 declaration mandatory; maximum, 80 ppm

f_1 in specific foodstuffs

g_1 in specific dietary products

h_1 maximum, 300 ppm

i_1 authorization of Ministry of Health required

j_1 licence issued by the Director of Food Administration; authorization of Ministry of Health required

k_1 maximum, 406 mg/l

l_1 only in low-calorie drinks; maximum, 1500 ppm; declaration mandatory

m_1 only in low-calorie foods

n_1 only in low-calorie drinks; maximum, 20,000 ppm; declaration mandatory

o_1 only in special dietetic products

p_1 caloric value not to exceed 80 kcal/l; special labelling mandatory

q_1 banned in powder form; special labelling mandatory

r_1 special labelling mandatory; maximum, 75 ppm

s_1 special labelling mandatory; maximum, 125 ppm

t_1 special labelling mandatory; maximum, 75 mg/l

u_1 only tablets allowed; special labelling mandatory

v_1 special regulations regarding advertising and purity of sweetener

w_1 only in dietetic products; special regulation to be followed

x_1 special regulations to be followed

y_1 special regulation to be followed; maximum, 0.8 g/l

z_1 approval of the National Board of Health and Consumer Interests required; special labelling mandatory

a_2 only in diabetic products; special labelling mandatory

b_2 medical prescription recommended; special labelling mandatory

c_2 only in dietetic products; government permission required prior to use

d_2 only in dietetic low-calorie products; maximum, 125 ppm

e_2 only in dietetic low-calorie products

f_2 special labelling mandatory; maximum, 100 mg/kg

g_2 only for diabetics; special labelling mandatory

h_2 allowed provisionally; maximum, 200 ppm

i_2 special labelling mandatory; not permitted in 'Bebida de extractos'

j_2 different maximum levels for different products

k_2 only in dietetic products; maximum, 0.5 g/kg, 0.5 g/l

l_2 special labelling mandatory; regulations regarding quantity limits to be followed

Reference

Hermes Sweeteners Ltd (1979) *International Legal Status of Saccharin and Cyclamate,* Zurich, Switzerland, February

THE MONOGRAPHS

(CYCLAMIC ACID, SODIUM CYCLAMATE, CALCIUM CYCLAMATE, CYCLOHEXYLAMINE & DICYCLOHEXYLAMINE)

I. Chemical and Physical Data

Cyclamic acid

1.1 Synonyms and trade names

Chem. Abstr. Services Reg. No.: 100-88-9

Chem. Abstr. Name: Cyclohexylsulfamic acid

Synonyms: Cyclamate; cyclohexanesulphamic acid; cyclohexylamidosulphuric acid; cyclohexylaminesulphonic acid; cyclohexylsulphamic acid; *N*-cyclohexylsulphamic acid

Trade names: Hexamic Acid; Sucaryl; Sucaryl Acid

1.2 Structural and molecular formulae and molecular weight

$C_6H_{13}NO_3S$ Mol. wt: 179.2

1.3 Chemical and physical properties of the pure substance

From Wade (1977) & Windholz (1976) unless otherwise specified

(a) Description: White crystalline powder with both an acid and a sweet taste

(b) Melting-point: 169-170°C

(c) Solubility: Soluble in water (1g in 7.5 ml), ethanol (1 in 3), acetone (1 in 7), chloroform (1 in 250), glycerol (1 in 12) and propylene glycol (1 in 4); insoluble in oils

(d) pH of 10% aqueous solution: 0.8-1.6 (Beck, 1969)

1.4 Technical products and impurities

In the US, cyclamic acid is available with a minimum purity of 98% on an anhydrous basis. The loss on drying at 105°C for 1 hr must not be more than 1% (Beck, 1969).

In the Federal Republic of Germany, cyclamic acid used as a food additive meets the following specifications: 98% active (on an anhydrous basis) and a maximum of 10 mg/kg cyclohexylamine, 1 mg/kg dicyclohexylamine, 1 mg/kg aniline and 30 mg/kg selenium (Bundesminister der Justiz, 1979).

Sodium cyclamate

1.1 Synonyms and trade names

Chem. Abstr. Services Reg. No.: 139-05-9

Chem. Abstr. Name: Cyclohexylsulfamic acid, monosodium salt

Synonyms: Cyclohexanesulphamic acid, monosodium salt; cyclohexylsulphamate sodium; cyclohexylsulphamic acid, monosodium salt; cyclamate sodium; sodium cyclohexanesulphamate; sodium cyclohexyl amidosulphate; sodium cyclohexylsul-phamate; sodium *N*-cyclohexylsulphamate; sodium cyclohexylsulphamidate

Trade names: Assugrin feinsuss; Assugrin vollsuss (also contains saccharin); Asugryn; Dulzor-Etas; Hachi-Sugar; Ibiosuc; Natreen (also contains saccharin); Sodium Sucaryl; Sucaryl sodium; Succaril (also contains saccharin); Sucrosa; Sucrun 7; Suessette; Suestamin; Sugarin; Sugaron

1.2 Structural and molecular formulae and molecular weight

$$CH_2 \underset{CH_2-CH_2}{\overset{CH_2-CH_2}{\diagup}} CH-N-\overset{\overset{O}{\|}}{\underset{\|}{S}}-O^- \ Na^+$$

$C_6H_{12}NNaO_3S$ Mol. wt: 201.2

1.3   Chemical and physical properties of the pure substance

From Wade (1977) and Windholz (1976)

(a)   *Description:*   White crystals or crystalline powder with an intensely sweet taste

(b)   *Solubility:*   Soluble in water (1g in 5 ml), ethanol (1 in 250) and propylene glycol (1 in 25); practically insoluble in chloroform and diethyl ether

(c)   *pH of a 10% aqueous solution:*   5.5-7.5

(d)   *Sweetness:*   Dilute aqueous solution is about 30 times sweeter than a solution containing an equal concentration by weight of sucrose

1.4   Technical products and impurities

In the US, sodium cyclamate was available commercially in 1970 as a US National Formulary (NF) grade crystalline powder containing 98-101% active ingredient on an anhydrous basis, a maximum of 30 mg/kg selenium, 25 mg/kg cyclohexylamine, 10 mg/kg heavy metals and 3 mg/kg arsenic. It was also available in: (1) aqueous solutions containing about 6% sodium cyclamate combined with about 0.6% sodium saccharin and (2) tablets containing about 50 mg sodium cyclamate combined with about 5 mg sodium saccharin (National Formulary Board, 1970).

In Canada, sodium cyclamate is available commercially as a crystalline powder containing 98-101% active ingredient on an anhydrous basis, a maximum of 30 mg/kg selenium, l0 mg/kg cyclohexylamine, 10 mg/kg heavy metals, 3 mg/kg arsenic and 0.5 mg/kg dicyclohexylamine.

In Western Europe, sodium cyclamate is available that meets the following specifications: 98-101% active ingredient on a dried basis and a maximum of 1% on drying, 10 mg/kg cyclohexylamine, 0.5 mg/kg dicyclohexylamine, 1 mg/kg aniline, 10 mg/kg heavy metals, 30 mg/kg selenium, 3 mg/kg arsenic, 500 mg/kg sulphate, 180 mg/kg chloride, 1 mg/kg dicyclohexylsulphamide, and no detectable barium.

In France, sodium cyclamate is available as a component of non-nutritive sweetening tablets containing 50 mg sodium cyclamate and 5 mg sodium saccharin.

In the Federal Republic of Germany, sodium cyclamate used as a food additive meets the following specifications: 98% active (on an anhydrous basis) and a maximum of 10 mg/kg cyclohexylamine, 1 mg/kg dicyclohexylamine, 1 mg/kg aniline and 30 mg/kg selenium (Bundesminister der Justiz, 1979).

Calcium cyclamate

1.1 Synonyms and trade names

Chem. Abstr. Services Reg. No.: 139-06-0

Chem. Abstr. Reg. Name: Cyclohexylsulfamic acid, calcium salt

Synonyms: Cyclamate calcium; calcium cyclohexane sulphamate; calcium cyclo-hexylsulphamate; cyclohexanesulphamic acid, calcium salt; cyclohexylsulphamic acid, calcium salt

Trade names: Cyclan; Cylan; Dietil; Sucaryl Calcium

1.2 Structural and molecular formulae and molecular weight

$C_{12}H_{24}CaN_2O_6S_2$ Mol. wt: 396.5

1.3 Chemical and physical properties of the pure substance

From Beck (1969) and National Formulary Board (1970)

(a) Description: White crystals or crystalline powder with an intensely sweet taste

(b) Solubility: Soluble in water (1g in 4 ml),ethanol (1 in 60) and propylene glycol (1 in 1.5); practically insoluble in benzene, chloroform and diethyl ether

(c) pH of aqueous solution: Neutral to litmus

(d) Sweetness: Similar to that of sodium cyclamate

1.4 Technical products and impurities

In the US, calcium cyclamate was available commercially in 1970 as a US National Formulary (NF) grade crystalline powder containing 98-101% active ingredient on an anhydrous basis, 6-9% water, a maximum of 30 mg/kg selenium, 25 mg/kg cyclohexylamine,

10 mg/kg heavy metals and 3 mg/kg arsenic. It was also available in: (1) aqueous solutions containing about 6% calcium cyclamate combined with about 0.6% calcium saccharin, and (2) tablets containing about 50 mg calcium cyclamate combined with about 5 mg calcium saccharin (National Formulary Board, 1970).

In Canada, calcium cyclamate is available commercially as a crystalline powder containing 98-101% active ingredient on an anhydrous basis, 6-9% water, a maximum of 30 mg/kg selenium, 10 mg/kg cyclohexylamine, 10 mg/kg heavy metals, 3 mg/kg arsenic and 0.5 mg/kg dicyclohexylamine.

In the Federal Republic of Germany, calcium cyclamate used as a food additive meets the following specifications: 98% active (on an anhydrous basis) and a maximum of 10 mg/kg cyclohexylamine, 1 mg/kg dicyclohexylamine, 1 mg/kg aniline and 30 mg/kg selenium (Bundesminister der Justiz, 1979).

Cyclohexylamine

1.1 Synonyms and trade names

Chem. Abstr. Services Reg. No.: 108-91-8

Chem. Abstr. Name: Cyclohexanamine

Synonyms: Aminocyclohexane; aminohexahydrobenzene; CHA; hexahydroaniline; hexahydrobenzenamine

1.2 Structural and molecular formulae and molecular weight

$$CH_2 \begin{array}{c} CH_2-CH_2 \\ \\ CH_2-CH_2 \end{array} CH-NH_2$$

$C_6H_{13}N$ Mol. wt: 99.2

1.3 Chemical and physical properties of the pure substance

From Carswell & Morrill (1937) and Windholz (1976) unless otherwise specified

(a) Description: Colourless liquid with a strong, fishy, amine odour

(b) Boiling-point: 134.5°C

(c)   *Crystallizing-point:* -17.7°C

(d)   *Density:* d_{25}^{25} 0.8647

(e)   *Refractive index:* n_{25}^{25} 1.4565

(f)   *Solubility:* Soluble in water and common organic solvents, including alcohols, ethers, ketones, esters, aliphatic and aromatic hydrocarbons and chlorinated hydrocarbons. Also soluble in oils such as mineral oil, peanut oil and soya bean oil (Abbott Laboratories, 1968)

(g)   *Reactivity:* Strong base. Forms salts with acids; reacts with (1) organic compounds containing an active halogen atom, (2) acid anhydrides and (3) alkylene oxides, to replace one or both hydrogen atoms on the nitrogen atom. Reacts with nitrous acid to form cyclohexanol (Abbott Laboratories, 1968).

1.4 Technical products and impurities

Cyclohexylamine is available commercially in the US as a colourless to slightly yellow liquid with the following typical specifications: purity, 98% minimum; density (25°C), 0.8645-0.8655; and 0.5% max by weight moisture content (Abbott Laboratories, 1968).

Cyclohexylamine is available in Japan as a clear liquid with the following specifications: purity, 99.7% min; moisture, 0.1% max; and distillation range 131.5-136°C.

Dicyclohexylamine

1.1 Synonyms and trade names

Chem. Abstr. Services Reg. No.: 101-83-7

Chem. Abstr. Name: *N*-Cyclohexylcyclohexanamine

Synonyms: Dodecahydrodiphenylamine; DCHA; *N,N*-dicyclohexylamine

1.2 Structural and molecular formulae and molecular weight

$$CH_2 \underset{CH_2-CH_2}{\overset{CH_2-CH_2}{\diagdown}} CH-NH-CH \underset{CH_2-CH_2}{\overset{CH_2-CH_2}{\diagup}} CH_2$$

$C_{12}H_{23}N$ Mol. wt: 181.3

1.3 Chemical and physical properties of the pure substance

From Carswell & Morrill (1937), unless otherwise specified

(a) *Description:* Colourless liquid with a faint fishy odour

(b) *Boiling-point:* 255.8 ^{o}C

(c) *Crystallizing-point:* -0.1^{o}C

(d) *Density:* d_{25}^{25} 0.9104

(e) *Refractive index:* n_d^{25} 1.4823

(f) *Solubility:* Only slightly soluble in water; soluble in all common organic solvents and miscible with cyclohexylamine

(g) *Reactivity:* Similar to cyclohexylamine, except that only monosubstitution products can be formed. Differs from cyclohexylamine in that it forms crystalline hydrates and alcohol complexes at low temperatures. Reacts with nitrous acid to form *N*-nitrosodicyclohexylamine (Rainey *et al.*, 1978)

1.4 Technical products and impurities

No data were available to the Working Group.

2. Production, Use, Occurrence and Analysis

2.1 Production and use

CYCLAMIC ACID, SODIUM CYCLAMATE AND CALCIUM CYCLAMATE

(a) Production

Cyclamic acid was synthesized by the reaction of barium-*N*-cyclohexylsulphamate (made by the sulphonation of cyclohexylamine with chlorosulphonic acid in chloroform followed by treatment with barium hydroxide) with sulphuric acid. Sodium cyclamate was synthesized by Sveda in 1937 (Beck, 1969) by the sulphonation of cyclohexylamine with chlorosulphonic acid in chloroform to produce cyclohexylammonium *N*-cyclohexyl-sulphamate, which was then treated with sodium hydroxide. Sodium cyclamate has also been made by the reaction of nitrocyclohexane with sodium dithionite in aqueous solution in the presence of trisodium phosphate (Audrieth & Sveda, 1944). Cyclamic acid has been manufactured in the US by the sulphonation of cyclohexylamine with sulphamic acid or sulphur trioxide. Sodium and calcium cyclamates have been prepared by neutralizing cyclamic acid with sodium hydroxide and calcium hydroxide, respectively, or by sulphonation of cyclohexylamine with sodium or calcium sulphamate (Beck, 1969).

Cyclamic acid, sodium cyclamate and calcium cyclamate were first produced commercially in the US in 1960 (US Tariff Commission, 1969), 1950 (US Tariff Commission, 1951) and 1953 (US Tariff Commission, 1954), respectively. Only one US company reported commercial production of an undisclosed amount (see preamble, p. 20) of each chemical in 1977 (US International Trade Commission, 1978a), all of which is believed to have been exported to European countries. However, prior to 1969, seven companies produced cyclamates. In 1968, an estimated 7400 thousand kg cyclamates were produced, compared with an estimated 770 thousand kg produced in 1957.

US imports of sodium cyclamate through principal US customs districts in 1969 were 21.3 thousand kg (US Tariff Commission, 1970); however, no imports have been reported recently.

Sodium and calcium cyclamates are produced by one company in the Federal Republic of Germany and by one in Spain.

Cyclamates are produced commercially in Taiwan and Brazil, but no information was available on the quantities produced. They have not been made commercially in Japan since about 1969. Prior to that data, an estimated 8130 thousand kg were produced annually, and 3250 thousand kg were exported annually.

(b) Use

The US consumption pattern for all three forms of cyclamates in 1965 was as follows: 53% in carbonated beverages, 17% in dry beverage bases, 13% in diet foods, 12% in sweetener formulations (e.g. , pharmaceutical products) and 5% in miscellaneous applications (e.g., toiletries) (Beck, 1969). Sodium and calcium cyclamates were used mainly in the form of the 10:1 cyclamate:saccharin salt mixture ((Wiegand, 1978).

Cyclamic acid itself (as opposed to its salts) was used in the US in the sweetening of effervescent tablets (Beck, 1969). Cyclamates have also been used in mouthwashes, toothpaste, lipsticks and paediatric drugs.

In the US, cyclamates were approved in the form of a New Drug Application for use as non-nutritive sweetening agents in early 1950. In the 1958 Food Additives Amendment to the Food, Drug, and Cosmetic Act, cyclamates were included among those substances that had been in use prior to 1958 and were then accorded GRAS (generally recognized as safe) status (Wiegand, 1978). On 21 October 1969, questions concerning the safety of cyclamates prompted the Food and Drug Administration (FDA) to remove cyclamates from GRAS status and to require that cyclamates intended for use in the dietary management of human disease must be relabelled to comply with drug provisions of the law and that existing stocks of artificially sweetened beverages and packaged mixes for the preparation of such beverages must be withdrawn from the market by 1 January 1970 (US Food & Drug Administration, 1969a). The FDA approved abbreviated new drug applications for cyclamates on 31 December 1969, provided certain labelling accompanied each end product (US Food & Drug Administration, 1969b). In the absence of adequate evidence of the safety of cyclamates, the FDA ruled that the continued sale of cyclamate-containing products with drug labelling would not be permitted as of 27 August 1970 (US Food & Drug Administration, 1970).

The Joint FAO/WHO Expert Committee on Food Additives established in 1967 (WHO, 1967) a temporary acceptable daily intake (ADI) of 50 mg/kg bw for total cyclamates. This was withdrawn in 1970 (WHO, 1971), and a temporary ADI of 4 mg/kg bw expressed as cyclamic acid was recommended in 1977 (WHO, 1977).

The regulatory status of non-nutritive sweeteners containing saccharin and/or cyclamates in various countries is outlined in the Appendix to the General Remarks on the Substances Considered, p. 39.

CYCLOHEXYLAMINE

(a) Production

Cyclohexylamine was synthesized in 1893 by Bayer by reduction of cyclohexanone oxime in absolute ethanol solution using metallic sodium (Carswell & Morrill, 1937). It is produced commercially in the US by: (1) the hydrogenation of aniline using cobalt-alumina catalysts; (2) ammonolysis of cyclohexyl chloride or cyclohexanol; and (3) reduction of nitrocyclohexane (Sandridge & Staley, 1978). In Japan, cyclohexylamine is produced commercially by two methods: (1) 63% is made by oxidation of cyclohexane to cyclohexanol followed by ammonolysis, and (2) 37% is made by the hydrogenation of aniline with nickel or cobalt catalysts.

Cyclohexylamine has been produced commercially in the US since 1936 (Carswell & Morrill, 1937). Three US companies reported production of 3115 thousand kg in 1977 (US International Trade Commission, 1978a), down from 5250 thousand kg in 1967 (US Tariff Commission, 1969). US imports through principal US customs districts in 1977 were 44.5 thousand kg (US International Trade Commission, 1978b).

Cyclohexylamine and its derivatives are produced by three companies each in the Federal Republic of Germany and the UK, and by one company in France and one in Italy.

It has been produced commercially in Japan since 1945. Three Japanese manufacturers reported production of 2500 thousand kg in 1977, up from 1300 thousand kg in 1974. Exports amounted to approximately 900 thousand kg in 1977, up from about 100 thousand kg in 1974.

(b) Use

Cyclohexylamine was used in the US in 1976 as follows: 55% in the production of rubber-processing chemicals, 30% in industrial water treatment, and 15% in miscellaneous applications (Anon., 1977).

The rubber-processing chemicals in which it is used include the vulcanization accelerator *N*-cyclohexyl-2-benzothiazolesulphenamide, of which 1858 thousand kg were produced in 1976 (Hancock, 1975; US International Trade Commission, 1977), and the antiozonant and antioxidant *N*-cyclohexyl-*N'*-phenyl-*para*-phenylenediamine, production of which is estimated to have been 900 thousand kg in 1976.

In industrial water treatment, cyclohexylamine is used as a corrosion inhibitor for binding of carbon dioxide in petroleum boiler systems (Nathan, 1965). Miscellaneous applications of cyclohexylamine are as a chemical intermediate in plasticizers, dyes (e.g., C.I. Acid Blue 62) (The Society of Dyers and Colourists, 1971), textile chemicals and, to a limited extent, in cyclamates (Hancock, 1975).

In western Europe, cyclohexylamine is used as an intermediate in the commercial production of the laurate, hydrobromide, hydrochloride, hydrofluoride, oleate, palmitate and stearate salts; rubber antiozonants and antioxidants; and others, such as 3-cyclo-hexylaminopropylamine and *N,N'*-dicyclohexylcarbodiimide.

In France, cyclohexylamine has been reported to be used in the manufacture of the herbicide, 3-cyclohexyl-5,6-trimethyleneuracil (Lenacil), which is used in horticulture and, primarily in Europe, on sugar beets, cereal grains and strawberries (Berg, 1979).

Of the estimated 1630 thousand kg cyclohexylamine used in Japan in 1977, approximately 77% was used to make rubber curing agents and 23% was used to make dyestuffs and as a corrosion inhibitor.

A major use of cyclohexylamine in the US was in the manufacture of sodium and calcium cyclamates until these products were banned from use in the US in 1970 (US Food & Drug Administration, 1970). In 1968, it was estimated that 60% of the total US demand of 7200 thousand kg cyclohexylamine was used in the production of cyclamates (Anon., 1968).

The US Food and Drug Administration has classified cyclohexylamine as safe for use in the preparation of steam that will be in contact with food, providing the concentration does not exceed 10 mg/kg in the steam and excluding its use in contact with milk and milk products (US Food & Drug Administration, 1978).

The American Conference of Governmental Industrial Hygienists (1978) approved a recommended threshold limit value of 10 ppm (40 mg/m^3) for skin exposure to cyclohexylamine in workroom air (in terms of an eight-hour time-weighted average).

The maximum acceptable concentration (MAC) in terms of ceiling value for occupational exposure to cyclohexylamine in the USSR in 1971 was reported to be 1 mg/m^3 (International Labour Organisation, 1971).

A temporary acceptable daily intake (ADI) of 50 mg/kg bw for total cyclamate was originally recommended by the joint FAO/WHO Expert Committee on Food Additives, then withdrawn, and later set at 4 mg/kg bw, expressed as cyclamic acid (WHO, 1977).

DICYCLOHEXYLAMINE

(a)   Production

Dicyclohexylamine was reported to be among the products formed when Sabatier & Senderens reduced aniline with hydrogen over a nickel catalyst in 1905 (Carswell & Morrill, 1937). It is believed to be produced commercially in the US by the vapour phase catalytic hydrogenation of aniline (Hancock, 1975).

In 1976, three US manufacturers reported production of dicyclohexylamine, and total sales amounted to 311 thousand kg (US International Trade Commission, 1977).

Only two companies reported production of an undisclosed amount (see preamble, p. 20) in 1977 (US International Trade Commission, 1978a). US imports through principal US customs districts were reported to be 43.2 thousand kg in that year (US International Trade Commission, 1978b).

In western Europe, dicyclohexylamine is produced by three companies in the Federal Republic of Germany and by two in the UK.

(b)   Use

Dicyclohexylamine is reportedly used as a chemical intermediate for the synthesis of a variety of derivatives used: (1) as corrosion inhibitors (e.g., to protect ferrous metal articles against atmospheric corrosion);   (2) as rubber-processing chemicals (e.g., the vulcanization accelerator, *N*-dicyclohexyl-2-benzothiazolesulphenamide);   and (3) in textiles, paints and varnishes (Hancock, 1975).

2.2 Occurrence

Cyclamic acid, sodium cyclamate, calcium cyclamate ,   cyclohexylamine and dicyclohexylamine are not known to occur as natural products; cyclohexylamine and dicyclohexylamine occur as metabolites of cyclamates (see section 3.2).

2.3 Analysis

Typical methods of analysis for the determination of cyclamic acid, sodium cyclamate and calcium cyclamate are summarized in Table 1. Methods for cyclohexylamine and dicyclohexylamine are summarized in Tables 2 and 3, respectively.

Table 1. Methods for the analysis of cyclamates

Sample matrix	Sample preparation	Assay procedure	Limit of detection	Reference
Bulk chemical	Treat with trifluoroacetic anhydride, dry, add internal standard (diphenyl in ethanol), centrifuge	GC/FID	-	Nagasawa et al., 1974
Bulk chemical	-	TLC	-	Guven & Savaskan, 1974
Pharmaceutical preparations	-	TLC	-	Nasierowska, 1975
Pharmaceutical preparations	-	TLC	3 µg	La Rotonda & Ferrara, 1975
Foods	-	TLC	3 µg	La Rotonda & Ferrara, 1975
Tinned seafood	Treat with chloranil and hydrogen peroxide	IDA/A (550 nm)	0.1 mg	Shimada et al., 1977

Abbreviations: GC/FID - gas chromatography/flame ionization detection; TLC - thin-layer chromatography; IDA/A - isotopic dilution analysis/absorptiometry

Table 2. Methods for the analysis of cyclohexylamine

Sample matrix	Sample preparation	Assay procedure	Limit of detection	Reference
Sodium cyclamate	Dissolve (hot water), cool, add sodium hydroxide (to pH 14), extract (dichloromethane), distill	GC/FID	-	Howard et al., 1969a
Calcium cyclamate	Dissolve (hot water), add EDTA solution, add sodium hydroxide (to pH 14), extract (dichloromethane), distill	GC/FID	-	Howard et al., 1969a
Food sweetener preparations	Wash (or dissolve in hot water if dry base), add EDTA solution[1], add sodium hydroxide (to pH 14), extract (dichloromethane), distill	GC/FID	-	Howard et al., 1969a
Water	-	Pol	-	Ivashchenko et al., 1975
Urine	Hydrolyse amines (reflux with hydrochloric acid), add sodium hydroxide (to pH 11.5), extract (dichloromethane), dry, extract (hydrochloric acid), add sodium hydroxide and sodium chloride, extract (n-hexane), add hydrochloric acid, sodium hydroxide, sodium chloride and n-hexane, agitate, centrifuge	GC/FID	0.1 μg/ml	Matsumura & Kohei, 1976

Abbreviations: GC/FID - gas chromatography/flame ionization detection; EDTA - ethylenediaminetetraacetic acid; Pol - polarography

[1] if the preparations contain calcium cyclamate

Table 3. Methods for the analysis of dicyclohexylamine

Sample matrix	Sample preparation	Assay procedure	Limit of detection	Reference
Sodium & calcium cyclamate	Liquid-liquid extraction (water, carbon tetrachloride, n-hexane)	GC/FID	-	Howard et al., 1969b
Sodium cyclamate	Dissolve (water), extract (chloroform), form bromophenol blue complex	VIS	1 mg/kg	Erskine & Williams, 1970

Abbreviations: GC/FID - gas chromatography/flame ionization detection; VIS - visible spectrometry

3. Biological Data Relevant to the
Evaluation of Carcinogenic Risk to Humans

3.1 Carcinogenicity studies in animals

CYCLAMIC ACID

No data were available to the Working Group.

SODIUM CYCLAMATE[1]

(a)   Oral administration in the drinking-water

Mouse: Groups of 60-80 mice of different strains were given commercial sodium cyclamate (source not stated; 99.5% pure) in drinking-water (6 g/l) for lifetime; the water intake was 3-4 ml/mouse per day, corresponding to 20-25 mg/mouse sodium cyclamate. In C3H male and female mice there were no differences in survival or in total tumour incidence between control and treated animals. In RIII males (the only sex treated) there were 3/22 lung tumours in treated animals and 0/19 in controls. Although lung tumours occurred in 3/16 untreated XVIIG female mice (the only sex tested), the incidence of such tumours was 16/20 in treated animals (P<0.001); one hepatocellular carcinoma and one mammary tumour also developed. Hepatocellular carcinomas were also seen in male F1(C3HxRIII) mice (the only sex tested); the incidence was 12/28 in controls and 22/34 in treated animals (P<0.05) (Rudali *et al.*, 1969) [The Working Group noted that a high proportion of animals was discarded. The conditions of animal husbandry were not reported, and it could not be ascertained whether histological examinations of all gross lesions had been undertaken. In addition, marked differences in mean survival times and time to appearance of first tumour make comparisons between strains difficult].

---

[1] The Working Group was aware of a study completed but not yet published on the carcinogenicity of sodium cyclamate in which hamsters were given the compound in drinking-water from 4 weeks before mating until delivery, the offspring being untreated (IARC, 1979).

Hamster: Groups of 30 male and 30 female random-bred Syrian golden hamsters received sodium cyclamate (Sigma Chemical Co., USA) containing 10 mg/kg cyclohexylamine at levels of 0, 0.156, 0.312, 0.625 and 1.25% in drinking-water for their natural life-span. The highest dose level used in this study was the maximum tolerated dose as determined in an 8-week study. The average daily consumption ranged from 47 mg/animal given the 0.156% level to 380 mg/animal given the 1.25% level. The mean survival time was 50-60 weeks in all groups, except those given 1.25% sodium cyclamate in which survival was 41 weeks. No apparent differences in tumour incidence were noted between treated and control animals. Bladders were examined histologically, and no bladder tumours were noted in any group (Althoff *et al.*, 1975) [The Working Group noted the limited reporting of the data and the short survival of the animals].

Monkey: Sodium cyclamate (source and purity unspecified) in aqueous solution was given orally at a dose level of 200 mg/kg bw per day, on 6 days a week to one male *Macaca mulatta* (rhesus) monkey for 6.4 years and to 2 females for 6.7 years. At those times, surviving monkeys were killed. Three animals of each sex served as controls. No evidence of hyperplastic or neoplastic changes was observed in any of the organs, including the urinary bladder (Coulston *et al.*, 1975, 1977) [The Working Group noted the small number of animals involved and the short duration of the observation period].

(b) Oral administration in the diet

Single-generation exposure

Mouse: Groups of 50 female Swiss mice received 0 or 5% sodium cyclamate (Abbott Laboratories, UK) in the diet for 18 months, at which time the survivors were killed. Average survival rates were not affected, and incidences of tumours of the forestomach, lung and liver and of lymphomas were similar in treated and control animals. No pathological alterations were observed macroscopically in the urinary bladder (Roe *et al.*, 1970) [The Working Group noted that the urinary bladders were not examined histologically].

Groups of 30 male and 30 female ASH-CS1 SPF mice received diets containing 0 (60 mice of each sex), 0.7, 1.75, 3.5 and 7.0% sodium cyclamate for 80 weeks; surviving animals (49, 23, 29, 23, 22 males; 45, 18, 20, 22, 16 females) were killed at between 80-84 weeks. The cyclamate (composite sample from Abbott Laboratories, Imperial Chemical Industries Ltd, and Laporte Industries Ltd, UK) reportedly contained less than 100 mg/kg cyclohexylamine. All bladders and tumours from all animals were examined microscopically, as were all tissues from those receiving 0 and 7.0%. In animals receiving the intermediate levels, microscopic examination was confined to the heart, liver, kidneys and any tissue that appeared abnormal at autopsy. Decreased weight gain and increased mortality were seen in cyclamate-treated females; a slight increase in the incidence of lymphosarcomas occurred in treated females (3/45 controls; 2/19 at 0.7, 3/18 at 1.75, 4/21 at 3.5 and 6/25 at 7.0%) ($P = 0.02$), and a lower incidence in treated males.

Additionally, a number of tumours were seen in treated animals that were not seen in controls (4 adenocarcinomas of the kidney in males, adenocarcinomas of the mammary gland in 1 male and 1 female and 4 reticulum-cell sarcomas in females), but their incidence was not statistically significant [P>0.05] (Brantom *et al.*, 1973).

Groups of 17, 38 and 33 female Charles River CD mice received sodium cyclamate (source and purity unspecified) in the diet at levels of 0, 1 or 5%, respectively, for up to 2 years. Animals that died before 6 months were not examined, and survival times were not reported. Animals were sacrificed when obvious tumours were seen or when they were moribund; all survivors were killed at 2 years. All animals that survived 6 months or longer were examined grossly, and any tissues with abnormal changes were examined histologically; in addition, all vital organs from at least 12 animals in each group were examined histologically. The incidences of total tumours (and in particular of vascular and lung tumours and lymphomas) were similar in treated and control groups (Homburger, 1978) [The Working Group noted the inadequate reporting of the experiment].

Rat: Weanling Osborne-Mendel rats were given sodium cyclamate (source and purity unspecified) in the diet at levels of 0, 0.01, 0.1, 0.5, 1.0 and 5% for 2 years. Each group consisted of 10 males and 10 females. Female animals receiving the 5% level gained less weight than the controls. Death rates during both the first and second years were equally distributed throughout all groups. No increased incidence of tumours compared with that in controls was reported (Fitzhugh *et al.*, 1951) [The Working Group noted the small number of animals in each group].

Sodium cyclamate (Abbott Laboratories, USA; purity unspecified) was administered in the diet to 7 male and 7 female weanling Osborne-Mendel rats per group at dose levels of 0.4, 2 and 10% for 101 weeks. A control group consisted of 28 animals. After 88 weeks, 3 transitional-cell papillomas of the urinary bladder were found: 1 in an animal receiving 0.4% and 2 in animals receiving 10% (sex unspecified). Occasionally, epithelial hyperplasia with atypia and parasitic infiltration (*Trichosomoides crassicauda*) were observed in the urinary bladder; nephrocalcinosis and renal calycine polyposis were also observed (Friedman *et al.*, 1972) [The Working Group noted the small number of animals examined histologically].

It was reported in an abstract that Osborne-Mendel rats (group size unspecified) were given sodium cyclamate (source and purity unspecified) at levels of 0.4, 2.0 and 10.0% in the diet for 20-23 months. Parasites of the urinary bladder (*Trichosomoides crassicauda*) were seen occasionally; none of the treated animals developed neoplastic lesions (Richardson *et al.*, 1972) (cf. calcium cyclamate) [The Working Group noted the incomplete reporting of this experiment. The apparently low number of survivors after 20 months (i.e., 19 controls), coupled with the presence of urinary bladder parasites, decreases the value of this study for the assessment of the carcinogenicity of cyclamates].

Two groups of 52 male and 52 female Sprague-Dawley rats received 0, 2 and 5% sodium cyclamate (Bayer-Werken AG, FRG) daily in the diet for up to 30 months, starting between 70 and 90 days of age, to give average total doses of 0, 882 and 2188 g/kg bw. The substance contained less than 4 mg/kg cyclohexylamine. At 24 months, approximately 10% of the animals were still alive. Sixteen percent of all animals had parasites (*Strongyloides capillaria*) in the urinary bladder. Histologically, fibromas, fibroadenomas or adenomas of the mammary gland (females) as well as thymomas (males) were found; the incidences were similar in all groups (5-7%). One urinary bladder papilloma was observed after 114 weeks in the group receiving 2% cyclamate (sex unspecified); and 1 transitional-cell carcinoma of the urinary bladder occurred simultaneously with multiple bladder stones in a male in the 2% cyclamate group that survived for 116 weeks (Schmähl, 1973).

It was reported in an abstract that groups of 54-56 male Wistar rats were fed 0 and 2.5 g/kg bw per day sodium cyclamate (source and purity unspecified) for up to 28 months. Ten to 16 rats of each group were killed at 12 months, 11 of each group at 24 months and all survivors (number unspecified) at 28 months. No urinary bladder tumours were observed (Furuya *et al.*, 1975) [The Working Group noted the incomplete reporting of this experiment].

A group of 95 male and 45 female Wistar SPF rats, aged 6-8 weeks at the start of the experiment, were fed for up to 2 years on a diet that provided 1.0 g sodium cyclamate/kg bw per day. A further group of 150 males and females were fed 2.0 g sodium cyclamate/kg bw per day. The sodium cyclamate (Abbott Laboratories, UK) contained 13 mg/kg cyclohexylamine. A control group of 55 male and 50 female Wistar SPF rats were maintained on a standard, cyclamate-free diet. The incidences of transitional-cell tumours of the bladder in surviving animals whose bladders were examined histologically were 0/98 in the control group, 1/84 in the group fed the lower dose of cyclamate and 2/143 in the group fed the higher dose (the sex of animals in which tumours occurred was not specified) (Hicks & Chowaniec, 1977; Hicks *et al.*, 1978).

Monkey: In a study in progress, now in its ninth year, monkeys of four different strains are treated with sodium cyclamate (Abbott Laboratories, USA) in the diet: 12 are given 100 mg/kg bw per day and 11 are given 500 mg/kg bw per day on 5 days a week. Clinical observation has failed to demonstrate any evidence of gross neoplasia (Sieber & Adamson, 1978) [The Working Group noted the small number of animals used and the fact that this study is not yet completed].

Multigeneration exposure

In the study reported here and in the other multigeneration studies cited below, animals of each sex of the parent generation were fed cyclamate from weaning (or very soon after weaning) throughout both pregnancy and the preweaning of their offspring. The offspring were placed on the same diet as their parents for their entire lifespan; thus, their exposure to cyclamate was increased by comparison with that of the Fo generation, by the length of the gestation and suckling periods.

Mouse: Sodium cyclamate (Bayer Farma NV, The Netherlands; 98-2-99.3% pure, containing 2.1 mg/kg cyclohexylamine) was fed continuously to Swiss SPF mice in a multigeneration study over 6 generations at levels of 0, 2 and 5%. The Fo, F3b and F6a generations, consisting of 50 males and 50 females, were used to study carcinogenicity. Each generation was treated for 84 weeks. Pathological alterations and urinary bladder calculi occurred with similar frequencies in control and treated groups. One transitional-cell carcinoma of the urinary bladder (grade II) occurred in a female of the F6a generation receiving 5% cyclamate. One anaplastic carcinoma of the urinary bladder was observed in a control female of the Fo generation (Kroes *et al.*, 1977).

(c)   Subcutaneous and/or intramuscular administration

Rat: Forty male and female albino Shell or Carworth Farm E rats (body weights, 100-150 g) were injected subcutaneously with 0.5 ml of a 15% aqueous solution of sodium cyclamate (Abbott Laboratories, UK; 99% pure) thrice weekly for 107 weeks. After 135 weeks (number of survivors unspecified), no tumours were found at the injection site (the only site reported) in treated animals (Grasso *et al.*, 1971) (cf. calcium cyclamate).

(d)   Other experimental systems

Bladder insertion (implantation): Sodium cyclamate (Abbott Laboratories, USA analytically pure)(4-5 mg) was mixed with 4 times its weight of cholesterol. Pellets containing sodium cyclamate were then inserted into the urinary bladder lumina in 2 separate trials using groups each of 100 female Swiss *mice* aged 60-90 days. Ninety-nine percent of the sodium cyclamate disappeared from the pellet within 7 hours. Identical groups received pellets of pure cholesterol. The experiment ran over 52 weeks, and only the bladders of animals surviving more than 25 weeks were examined microscopically. The first urinary bladder carcinoma was seen in a cyclamate-treated animal 33 weeks after surgical implantation. The overall incidences were 45/58 (trial 1) and 30/49 (trial 2) for cyclamate-treated mice, as compared with 8/63 (trial 1) and 5/43 (trial 2) for animals exposed to pure cholesterol pellets (P<0.001). The carcinomas in cyclamate-exposed mice were more frequently multiple, invaded the muscle more frequently, had a higher mitotic index and showed more squamous and glandular metaplastic changes than those in tumour-bearing controls. In no other tissues was there a tumour incidence different from that in control mice (Bryan & Ertürk, 1970) (cf. sodium saccharin, p. 139).

(e) Administration in conjunction with known carcinogens

Benzo(a)pyrene (BP): Groups of 50 female Swiss *mice* received an initial single gastric instillation of 0.2 ml polyethylene glycol either alone or containing 50 µg BP (purities unspecified). Seven days later, the test diet, containing 5% sodium cyclamate (Abbott Laboratories, UK) was fed for 72 weeks. Average survival rates were no different from those in controls. Although mice treated with BP showed an increased incidence of papillomas of the forestomach (20/61), cyclamate did not enhance the occurrence (4/41). Hepatocellular adenomas, pulmonary neoplasms and malignant lymphomas occurred with similar frequencies in all groups. No pathological alterations were observed macroscopically in the urinary bladder (Roe *et al.*, 1970) [The Working Group noted that BP is not organotropic for the bladder and that the urinary bladders were not examined histologically].

Butyl-4-butanolnitrosamine (BBN): Groups of 40 male 3-month-old Sprague-Dawley *rats* received the following treatments: group 1, control. group 2, 10 mg/kg bw BBN (synthesized in the authors' laboratory) in the drinking-water daily for life; group 3, the same dose of BBN plus 2.5 g/kg bw per day sodium cyclamate (Farbenfabriken Bayer, FRG; containing less than 2 mg/kg cyclohexylamine) in the diet. The average total doses were 3.29 g/kg BBN and 805 g/kg bw sodium cyclamate. After an average induction time of 400 ± 45 days, all 40 animals treated with BBN died with squamous-cell carcinomas of the urinary bladder. Of animals fed the combination diet, 27/29 rats developed typical bladder carcinomas and 2 showed extensive papillomatosis without histological indications of malignant transformations; the 11 still alive at the time the report was published had haematuria, indicating the presence of urothelial lesions (Schmähl & Krüger, 1972) [The study when reported was still in progress. The presence of bladder tumours in all rats given only BBN precluded the possibility that an enhancement could be demonstrated with cyclamate].

2-Acetylaminofluorene (AAF): The combined effect of sodium cyclamate (Abbot Laboratories, USA) and AAF was studied in groups of 12 female Horton-Sprague-Dawley *rats*: group 1, control; group 2, 300 mg AAF/kg diet; and group 3, 300 mg AAF/kg diet + 5% sodium cyclamate. The experiment was terminated at 40 weeks. The combined incidences of mammary and ear-duct tumours were: group 1, 0/12; group 2, 11/12; group 3, 2/12. Hepatocellular adenomas were found in all rats fed AAF. All rats fed AAF with or without cyclamate demonstrated microscopic bladder hyperplastic lesions; none of the animals developed neoplastic lesions of this organ. The controls developed no tumours (Ershoff & Bajwa, 1974) [The Working Group noted the inadequate number of animals, the weight loss and the fact that food consumption was not measured, so that it was not possible to assess the intake of AAF or cyclamate].

N-*Nitroso*-N-*methylurea (NMU)*: A group of 30 female Wistar SPF *rats*, 6-8 weeks of age, were pretreated with 1.5 mg NMU, then 2 days later were fed 1.0 g sodium cyclamate/kg bw per day for life or up to 2 years; 50 further females were pretreated with 1.5 mg NMU and then fed 2.0 g sodium cyclamate/kg bw per day. The sodium cyclamate (Abbott Laboratories, UK) contained 13 mg/kg cyclohexylamine; NMU (purity unspecified) was dissolved in 0.9% sodium chloride (pH 7.0) and instilled into the bladder. Control groups consisted of 55 male and 50 female untreated rats, groups of 95 male and female rats fed 1.0 g sodium cyclamate/kg bw per day and 150 males and females fed 2.0 g sodium cyclamate/kg bw per day. For concurrent NMU controls, 85 females were given 1.5 mg NMU, and 50 were given 2.0 mg NMU and maintained on a cyclamate-free diet for 2 years. The incidences of transitional-cell neoplasms of the bladders in surviving animals whose bladders were examined histologically were: untreated controls, 0/98; lower dose of sodium cyclamate alone, 1/84; higher dose of sodium cyclamate alone, 2/143; NMU-treated animals (1.5 and 2.0 mg), 0/124; 1.5 mg NMU followed by the lower dose of sodium cyclamate, 14/24 (58%); 1.5 mg NMU followed by the higher dose of sodium cyclamate, 20/45 (44%; P<0.0005). The first bladder tumour was seen after 87 weeks in the cyclamate-fed control group and after 8 weeks in the NMU-initiated and sodium cyclamate-fed test groups (Hicks *et al.*, 1978).

A single dose of 2 mg NMU (German Cancer Research Centre, FRG) in 0.5 ml distilled water was instilled into the urinary bladder of 50 female Wistar *rats* (AF-Han strain; body weight, 195 g). Thereafter, the animals were given 2% sodium cyclamate (Abbott Laboratories, USA; purity unspecified), increased after 10 weeks to 4%, in the diet for life (1.4-2.4 g/kg bw per day). Control groups consisted of 100 untreated female rats, 50 females receiving NMU alone and 50 females receiving distilled water. A further group of 50 female rats treated with NMU were given 3% calcium carbonate in the diet instead of sodium cyclamate. Survival at two years was: controls, 59/100; water controls, 28/50; NMU-treated, 13/50; NMU + calcium carbonate-treated, 15/50; NMU + sodium cyclamate treated, 14/50. In the NMU-treated groups, the first tumour of the urinary bladder was found after 14 weeks. Urothelial neoplasms (benign and malignant) occurred in the renal pelvis, ureter and urinary bladder. The overall incidences of urinary tract tumours were 57% (NMU alone; survival 76 ± 29 weeks), 70% (NMU + cyclamate; survival, 81 ± 27 weeks) and 65% (NMU + calcium carbonate; survival, 86 ± 23 weeks). In the renal pelvis, frequencies were 28, 43 and 43%; the ureter showed incidences of 17, 6 and 11%; and the urinary bladder had frequencies of 39, 40 and 39%, respectively. Calcifications in the urinary tract, including stone formation, were similar in all treated groups, including water controls; they did not correlate with tumour occurrences. One tumour of the urinary tract was seen in the untreated controls and one in controls receiving a water instillation into the urinary bladder (Mohr *et al.*, 1978) [The Working Group noted that many tumours were found, and that the animals were heavier than those used in the experiment by Hicks *et al.*, 1978] .

SODIUM CYCLAMATE/SACCHARIN MIXTURES

(a)   Oral administration in the diet

Single-generation exposure

Rat: Two groups of 52 male and 52 female Sprague-Dawley rats, between 70 and 90 days of age, were given a 10:1 mixture of sodium cyclamate:sodium saccharin (Bayer-Werken AG, FRG) daily in the diet for up to 30 months. The cyclamate in the mixture contained less than 4 mg/kg cyclohexylamine. The mixture was administered at doses of 2 and 5%. An identical group served as controls. At 24 months, approximately 10% of the initial number of animals were still alive. Except for the occurrence of bladder parasites (*Strongyloides capillaria*) in 16% of animals, all examinations were negative. A similar frequency of benign neoplasms occurred in all groups (fibromas, fibroadenomas or adenomas of the mammary gland in females and thymomas in males) (Schmähl, 1973).

It was reported in an abstract that two groups of 54-56 male Wistar rats received 0 or 2.5 g/kg bw per day of a mixture of sodium cyclamate:sodium saccharin (10:1) (source and purity unspecified) in the diet for 28 months. Ten to 16 rats of each group were killed at 12 months, 11 at 24 months and all survivors at 28 months. No treated or control animals developed tumours of the urinary bladder (Furuya *et al.*, 1975) [The Working Group noted the incomplete reporting of this experiment].

Groups of 35 male and 45 female FDRL strain Wistar-derived weanling rats were fed a 10:1 mixture of sodium cyclamate:saccharin (Abbott Laboratories, USA; purity and method of manufacture unspecified) in the diet at doses of 0, 500, 1120 and 2500 mg/kg bw per day for 2 years. From week 79 the original dose groups were split, and 50% of the survivors in each group, except the untreated controls, received in addition cyclohexylamine hydrochloride in the diet. The 500 mg group received 25 mg, the 1120 mg group 56 mg, and the 2500 mg group received 125 mg cyclohexylamine/kg bw per day. Mortality rates were similar in control and test groups. Treatment-related pathological changes were seen only in the kidney and bladder. Pelvic hyperplasia was observed more often in the treated groups (8/80, 21/80 and 16/80, as compared with 3/80 in controls). Among animals surviving more than 49 weeks, 9/25 male and 3/35 female rats at the 2500 mg/kg bw dose, compared with 0/35 and 0/45 female controls, developed transitional-cell carcinomas of the urinary bladder. Of these, 3 male and 2 female rats had received cyclohexylamine. Two of the bladder carcinoma-bearing animals had calculi; 18 rats at this dose level had nonmalignant proliferative bladder lesions. In the lower dose groups, nonmalignant proliferative lesions were found, but their incidence was not significantly higher than that in controls. Renal calcification was seen in 7/12 rats with bladder carcinomas; *Trichosomoides crassicauda* infection was present in one rat with bladder cancer and 4 rats with nonneoplastic proliferative lesions at the highest dose level, in 4 given the 1120 mg/kg dose, in 2 given the 500 mg/kg dose and in 5 control animals (Oser *et al.*, 1975; Price *et al.*, 1970).

Multigeneration exposure

Mouse: In a multigeneration study, a 10:1 mixture of sodium cyclamate:saccharin (5 or 2% and 0.5 or 0.2%, respectively; Bayer Farma NV, The Netherlands) was fed continuously to Swiss SPF mice over 6 generations. The cyclamate was 98.2-99.3% pure and contained 2.1 mg/kg cyclohexylamine; the saccharin contained 0.5% *ortho*-toluenesulphonamide. The Fo (parental), F3b and F6a generations, consisting of 50 males and 50 females each, were used for the carcinogenicity studies and were treated for 84 weeks. Pathological alterations and urinary bladder calculi occurred with similar frequencies in control and treated groups. Four neoplasms of the urinary bladder occurred: three anaplastic carcinomas (1 in a female control of the Fo generation and 2 in females of the Fo and F6a generations fed 2% cyclamate plus 0.2% saccharin) and one papilloma (in a male of the F6a generation given 2% cyclamate plus 0.2% saccharin). The mean latent period was more than 80 weeks (Kroes *et al.*, 1977).

CALCIUM CYCLAMATE

(a)   Oral administration in the drinking-water

Hamster: Groups of 30 male and 30 female random-bred Syrian golden hamsters received calcium cyclamate (Sigma Chemical Co., USA) containing a trace of cyclohexylamine at levels of 0, 0.156, 0.312, 0.625 and 1.25% in drinking-water for their natural lifespan. The highest dose level used in this study was the maximum tolerated dose as determined in an 8-week study. The average daily consumption ranged from 38 mg per animal given the 0.156% level to 311 mg per animal given the 1.25% level. The mean survival time was 50-60 weeks in all groups, except those given 0.625% (43 weeks) and 1.25% (29 weeks). No apparent differences in tumour incidence were noted between treated and control animals. Bladders were examined histologically, and no bladder tumours were noted in any group (Althoff *et al.*, 1975) [The Working Group noted the limited reporting of the data and the short survival of the animals].

(b)   Oral administration in the diet

Single-generation exposure

Rat: Male Holtzman rats (20-28 per group) received a normal (20%) or low (10%) protein semisynthetic diet containing 0, 1 or 2% calcium cyclamate (City Chemical Corp., USA) for 75 weeks. A transitional-cell papilloma occurred in the urinary bladder of 1/11 animals examined (20% protein, 2% calcium cyclamate diet); the kidneys and urinary bladder of this animal contained stones and calcium deposits. In a simultaneous investigation, 0.4, 2 or 10% calcium cyclamate (Abbott Laboratories, USA) was given with the normal chow diet to 14 male and 14 female Osborne-Mendel rats for 101 weeks. A control group consisted of 28 animals. After 88 weeks, 2 transitional-cell papillomas of the urinary bladder (1/6 in the 0.4% group and 1/4 in the 10% group) were noted; 3 transitional-cell carcinomas of the urinary bladder were also found (2/6 in the 0.4% group and 1/4 in the 10% group). Some animals in this study had bladder parasites (Friedman *et al.*, 1972) [The Working Group noted the small number of surviving animals].

It was reported in an abstract that Osborne-Mendel rats (group size unspecified) were given calcium cyclamate (source and purity unspecified) at levels of 0.4, 2.0 and 10% in the diet for 20-23 months. Three of 23 rats treated for 20 months developed invasive transitional-cell carcinomas of the urinary bladder; and one bladder carcinoma occurred among 4 rats fed the 10% level and 2 among 6 rats fed the 0.4% level. Urinary bladder calculi also occurred in 2 animals with urinary bladder tumours. Parasites *(Trichosomoides crassicauda)* were not seen in tumour-bearing animals but occurred in other animals in the study (Richardson *et al.*, 1972) (cf. sodium cyclamate) [The apparently low number of survivors after 20 months (i.e., 19 controls), coupled with the presence of urinary bladder parasites, decreases the value of this study for the assessment of the carcinogenicity of cyclamates].

Multigeneration exposure

Rat: In a 2-generation study reported as an abstract, calcium cyclamate (5%, source and purity unspecified) was fed to Charles River CD rats. The animals were allowed to mate to produce two litters. Serial sacrifices were performed at 14 and 18 months; 48 male and 48 female Fla weanling offspring were selected from each group and were continued on the same test regimen as their parents. The study was continued until the number of survivors in a group was 20% of the starting number. The last rats were killed 28 months after the first weanlings were selected for the chronic study. There were no significant differences between test and control groups regarding survival. Histological examination of urinary bladders from rats surviving longer than 18 months showed no neoplasms (Taylor & Friedman, 1974).

(c)   Subcutaneous and/or intramuscular administration

Rat: Male and female albino Shell or Carworth Farm E rats (body weights, 100-150 g) were injected subcutaneously with an aqueous solution of calcium cyclamate (Abbott Laboratories, UK; 99% pure) thrice weekly. One ml of a 5% solution given for 85 weeks induced fibrosarcomas at the site of injection in 4/10 surviving rats after 66 weeks of treatment (20 animals initially, remaining animals killed at 85 weeks), whereas 0.5 ml of a 15% solution given for 107 weeks caused fibrosarcomas at the site of injection in 14/24 rats alive after 49 weeks of treatment (30 animals initially, remaining animals killed after 135 weeks) (Grasso *et al.*, 1971) (cf. sodium cyclamate).

CYCLOHEXYLAMINE

(a)   Oral administration

Single-generation exposure

Mouse: Groups of 50 female and 48 male weanling ASH-CS1 SPF mice received cyclohexylamine hydrochloride (Laporte Industries Ltd, UK;   purity unspecified) in the regular diet at levels of 0, 300, 1000 or 3000 mg/kg of diet for 80 weeks.   The experiment was terminated between 80 and 84 weeks, at which time a similar survival rate was observed among all groups.   The numbers of mice with tumours occurring at all sites were 16/46 (control), 14/45 (300 mg/kg), 10/31 (1000 mg/kg) and 11/46 (3000 mg/kg) males; and 11/44 (control), 15/46 (300 mg/kg), 15/42 (1000 mg/kg) and 10/44 (3000 mg/kg) females.   No statistical differences in the incidences of the main types of tumours were observed among the various groups.   Some mice developed tumours not seen in controls, but these were considered to be sporadic findings and within the normal range of spontaneous tumours found in this strain of mice (Hardy *et al.*, 1976).

Rat: Cyclohexylamine (Voroshilov Scientific Research Institute for Organic By-Products and Dyes, USSR;   chemically pure) was given to 22 male and 28 female rats (strain unspecified) with the food at a rate of 0.5 ml of a 5% solution of cyclohexylamine in sunflower oil on 6 days per week for 52 weeks (total dose, 8925 mg/animal).   After 18 months, 20 rats were still alive, and none had tumours, although livers and kidneys showed degenerative changes.   In 130 rats considered to be controls, which had been injected subcutaneously with octadecylamine or methylstearylamine for 10 months and had survived 20 months, no tumours were detected (Pliss, 1958) [The Working Group noted the absence of tumours in the group considered to be controls].

Cyclohexylamine sulphate (Abbott Laboratories, USA) was fed to 25 male and 25 female Charles River albino rats for 2 years at doses of 0, 0.15, 1.5 and 15 mg/kg bw per day.   After 104 weeks, 13-16 animals were still alive in the 0.15 and 1.5 mg/kg bw groups and 8 males and 9 females in the 15 mg/kg bw group.   An invasive transitional-cell carcinoma of the bladder was observed in 1/8 male survivors of the high-dose group.   No other relevant findings were noted (Price *et al.*, 1970).

Cyclohexylamine (Bayer-Werken AG, FRG;   purity unspecified) was fed to 52 male and 52 female Sprague-Dawley rats aged 70-90 days at a daily dose of 200 mg/kg bw (average total dose, 177 g/kg bw) for 30 months.   A group of the same size served as untreated controls.   Sixteen percent of all animals had bladder parasites (*Strongyloides capillaria*).   The incidences of benign and malignant tumours were similar in treated and control animals (Schmähl, 1973).

Five groups of 30 male and 30 female FDRL weanling rats were given 0, 15, 50, 100 and 150 mg/kg bw cyclohexylamine hydrochloride (Baker grade) in the diet for 2 years. At the end of the second year, 46% of controls and 45.1 and 55% of treated males and females were still alive. A few tumours occurred in all groups, with similar incidence, location and characteristics. Mucosal thickening of the bladder was seen in animals given the 50 and 150 mg levels; no neoplasms of the urinary bladder were observed. *Trichosomoides crassicauda* was present in all rats surviving more than 65 weeks (Oser *et al.*, 1976).

Groups of 48 male and 48 female Wistar SPF rats were fed diets containing 0, 600, 2000 or 6000 mg/kg diet cyclohexylamine hydrochloride (Laporte Industries Ltd, UK) for 2 years. Average intake was 24, 82 and 300 mg/kg bw per day for males and 35, 120 and 440 mg/kg bw per day for females. Rats still alive at week 104 were killed: these comprised 24, 27, 30 and 43 males and 32, 38, 44 and 41 females. A dose-related reduction in body weight gain was observed throughout the study. Most tumours occurred with a similar frequency in treated and control rats; however, a few tumours were found in the treated animals which did not occur in controls, but these were distributed randomly, and their incidence was not significantly different. Total tumour occurrence was not different among the groups (Gaunt *et al.*, 1976).

Multigeneration exposure

In a multigeneration study, 0.5% cyclohexylamine sulphate (Bayer-Werken AG, FRG; purity unspecified) was administered continuously to groups of Swiss SPF mice in the diet for 84 weeks. The Fo, F3b and F6a generations, consisting of 50 males and 50 females, were used for carcinogenicity studies. There were no differences in tumour incidences between treated and control animals. One female control animal developed an anaplastic carcinoma of the urinary bladder at 82 weeks. Urinary bladder calculi were observed in all groups (Kroes *et al.*, 1977).

DICYCLOHEXYLAMINE

(a)   Oral administration

Rat: Groups of 25 male and 25 female rats (strain unspecified) received multiple s.c. injections of 30 mg dicyclohexylamine (Voroshilov Scientific Research Institute for Organic By-Products and Dyes, USSR; chemically pure) for 8 weeks. At this time, necrosis developed at the injection site, and the treatment was continued by feeding a diet supplemented with a dose of 0.5 ml of a 5% solution in sunflower oil, 6 times a week for 52 weeks (total dose, 8875 mg). One hepatic neoplasm developed after 84 weeks and 1 sarcoma of the omentum after 90 weeks (Pliss, 1958) [The Working Group noted the inadequacy of the reporting of the data and the lack of appropriate controls].

Groups of 17 male and 13 female rats (strain unspecified) received dicyclohexy-lamine nitrite (Voroshilov Scientific Research Institute for By-Products and Dyes, USSR; chemically pure) in the diet at a level of 1 ml in a 3% aqueous solution on 6 days a week for 12 months (total dose, 9180 mg). After 17 months, one rat showed a mesenteric sarcoma (Pliss, 1958) [The Working Group noted the lack of concurrent controls].

(b)   Subcutaneous and/or intramuscular administration

Mouse: Groups of 22 male and 35 female strain 'D' mice (obtained by crossing CC_{57} white with C_{57} black) received daily s.c. injections of 0.05 ml of a 2.6% solution of dicyclo-hexylamine in sunflower oil (Voroshilov Scientific Research Institute for Organic By-Products and Dyes, USSR; chemically pure) for a total of 11-12.5 months (total dose, 60.1-79.3 mg). Among 15 mice (sex unspecified) that lived more than 12 months, 4 developed sarcomas at the site of injection (Pliss, 1958) [The Working Group noted the ab-sence of solvent-treated controls].

Groups of 31 male and 23 female strain 'D' mice were given daily s.c. injections of 0.1 ml of a 1% aqueous solution of dicyclohexylamine nitrite (Voroshilov Scientific Research Institute for By-Products and Dyes, USSR; chemically pure) over 12-13 months. Among 23 mice (sex unspecified) that lived more than 12 months, 5 developed neoplasms: 2 hepatocellular adenomas, one papillary cystadenoma of the lung, one papillary adenoma of the lung and one cavernous haemangioma of the liver (Pliss, 1958) [The Working Group noted the absence of solvent-treated controls].

Rat: Dicyclohexylamine nitrite (Voroshilov Scientific Research Institute for By-Products and Dyes, USSR; chemically pure) was administered subcutaneously to 34 male and 22 female rats (strain unspecified) at a level of 0.5 ml of a 2% aqueous solution weekly. Among 31 rats (sex unspecified) that lived more than 12 months, 7 developed tumours at various sites (Pliss, 1958) [The Working Group noted the inadequacy of the reporting of the data and the lack of appropriate controls].

3.2   Other relevant biological data

Biological data on cyclamates and cyclohexylamine have been reviewed (WHO, 1967, 1971, 1977).

(a)   Experimental systems

Toxic effects

Cyclamates

The LD_{50} of sodium cyclamate by oral administration to mice and rats is between 10 and 12 g/kg bw (Richards *et al.*, 1951); the oral LD_{50} in male and female hamsters is 9.8

and 12.2 g/kg bw, respectively;   for calcium cyclamate, the respective values were 4.5 and 6 g/kg bw (Althoff *et al.*, 1975).   Following i.v. injection of sodium cyclamate, the LD_{50} values were 4 g/kg bw for mice and 3.5 g/kg bw for rats (Richards *et al.*, 1951).

Oral doses of 2 or 3 g/kg bw sodium cyclamate to cats caused occasional vomiting (Richards *et al.*, 1951).   Dogs given 2 or 4 g/kg bw sodium cyclamate orally daily for 30 days showed no significant toxic effects (Taylor *et al.*, 1968).

In a six-generation experiment with Swiss mice receiving 2 or 5% sodium cyclamate (purity 98.2-99.3%, 2.1 mg/kg cyclohexylamine) in their diet, no toxicity was observed. No histopathological alterations due to treatment were found in long-term studies (21 months) performed with the third and sixth generations (Kroes *et al.*, 1977).

It was reported in an abstract that degeneration and loss of seminiferous epithelium of the testis were seen in male rats given 2.5 g/kg bw per day sodium cyclamate in the diet for 28 months (Furuya *et al.*, 1975).

I.p. injection of up to 500 mg/kg bw calcium cyclamate for 5 days did not increase the incidence of morphological sperm abnormalities in mice (Wyrobek & Bruce, 1975).

Addition of 5 or 10% calcium cyclamate to the diet of rats for 8 weeks increased water consumption and reduced the growth rate of both males and females; it increased the weight of the adrenals in animals of both sexes;   the testes showed atrophy and degeneration of the seminiferous tubules (Nees & Derse, 1967).

Testicular atrophy was observed in rats given 2500 mg/kg bw per day of a 10:1 mixture of sodium cyclamate:sodium saccharin (Oser *et al.*, 1975).

Diarrhoea was observed in dogs receiving 1.5 g/kg bw per day sodium cyclamate (Löser, 1977) and in rats receiving 5% sodium cyclamate in the diet (Fitzhugh *et al.*, 1951) or 10% calcium cyclamate in the diet (Nees & Derse, 1967).   The laxative action of cyclamates in dogs, rats and mice is similar to that of sulphates (Hwang, 1966).

Prolonged administration of 2% sodium cyclamate in drinking-water to guinea-pigs caused changes in liver, kidney and pancreatic cells (Hagmüller *et al.*, 1969).   In a subchronic study, 5-week-old mice were given 0, 1, 2, 4, 8 and 16% calcium cyclamate in drinking-water for 5 weeks.   Levels of 8 and 16% significantly reduced survival and body weight; body weight was slightly reduced with the 4% level.   Microscopic vacuolated cells were observed in the liver parenchyma and renal tubules, especially in animals treated with the lower levels. Desquamatous changes and necrosis occurred in the transitional epithelium of the urinary bladder (Toth, 1972).   It was reported in an abstract that monkeys given single doses of 4 or 8 g/kg bw or rats given 5 daily doses of 2-8 g/kg bw sodium cyclamate orally showed 'diffuse mild vesiculation' of the endoplasmic reticulum associated with vacuolization of livers and kidneys (Stein *et al.*, 1967).

Sodium cyclamate caused a reduction in blood clotting ability in rabbits (Göttinger *et al.*, 1968). A level of 5% in the diet of rats reduced survival and weight gain to a greater extent when the major dietary carbohydrate was sucrose or glucose than when it was corn starch (Ershoff, 1977). These effects could be reduced by addition of the anion-exchange resin cholestyramine to the diet (Ershoff, 1976). The repeated oral administration of 3 g/kg bw calcium cyclamate to female hamsters caused myocardial lesions, including coronary sclerosis, calcification and necrosis of skeletal muscle and nephrocalcinosis (Bajusz, 1969).

The administration of 5% calcium cyclamate in drinking-water to rabbits for 150 days delayed and suppressed the titre of antibodies against bovine serum albumin (Hampton & Myers, 1976). Prolonged administration of calcium cyclamate to rats reduced the activity of enzymes in the intestinal mucosa, including acid and alkaline phosphatase, ATP-ase and enzymes involved in glycolysis, the Krebs cycle and in protein and lipid metabolism (Bernier *et al.*, 1968).

Cyclohexylamine

Cyclohexylamine is about 10 times more toxic than cyclamate: the LD_{50} by i.p. injection in mice is 620 mg/kg bw and in rats about 350 mg/kg bw; the LD_{50} in dogs following i.v. injection is about 200 mg/kg bw (Miyata *et al.*, 1969).

In a six-generation experiment with Swiss mice receiving 0.5% cyclohexylamine sulphate (containing several unspecified impurities, of which the major one was 0.5% *ortho*-toluenesulphonamide) in the diet, reduced body weight was found in all 6 generations and was especially pronounced in the first generations and in females. Food intake, as measured in the sixth generation, was normal. No histopathological changes were found in the various organs tested (Kroes *et al.*, 1977).

Feeding a diet containing 600 to 6000 mg/kg of diet cyclohexylamine hydrochloride to rats for 13 weeks (Gaunt *et al.*, 1974) or for 2 years (Gaunt *et al.*, 1976) resulted in reduced food and water consumption in animals receiving the highest dose and in impaired weight gain in males at 2000 and 6000 mg/kg of diet and in females at 600-6000 mg/kg of diet. The relative weights of a number of organs (brain, spleen, kidney and stomach) were reduced after 2 years of treatment of males with 6000 mg/kg. Although there was a reduction of the absolute weight of the testes after 2 years of treatment with 6000 mg/kg, the relative weight was normal after 2 years or slightly reduced (P=0.01-0.05) after 13 weeks of treatment. Histologically, a bilateral atrophy of the testes was noted in animals at the 2000 and 6000 mg/kg levels after 13 weeks of feeding (P=0.0l-0.05), but after 2 years of treatment this effect was only pronounced in the group receiving 6000 mg/kg. Reproduction was found to be normal under these conditions.

Feeding rats 2 and 6 g/kg of diet cyclohexylamine hydrochloride for 90 days led to reduced growth rate; reduced testis weight and spermatogenesis were observed with the highest dose (Mason & Thompson, 1977). Testicular atrophy was observed in rats fed 50 and 150 mg/kg bw (Oser et al., 1976).

I.v. injections of small doses (0.4-3.7 mg/kg bw) of cyclohexylamine increased the arterial pressure and pulse rate in rats, guinea-pigs and cats (Classen et al., 1968). Coadministration of monoamine oxidase inhibitors did not potentiate the effect on blood pressure in cats (Yamamura et al., 1968). Oral administration of doses up to 150 mg/kg bw cyclohexylamine hydrochloride to rats had no sympathomimetic activity (Bailey et al., 1972).

Dicyclohexylamine

The oral LD_{50} of dicyclohexylamine in rats is 373 mg/kg bw (Marhold et al., 1967). The oral LD_{50} of dicyclohexylamine nitrite in mice was 205 mg/kg bw (Pliss, 1958).

S.c. injection of 0.12 mg dicyclohexylamine per mouse produced convulsions immediately after administration (Pliss, 1958).

Teratogenicity and embryotoxicity

Cyclamates

Oral administration of 50-250 mg/kg bw per day sodium cyclamate over the total organogenesis phase to mice (Lorke, 1969a), rats (Fritz & Hess, I968) and rabbits (Klotzsche, 1969) gave no indication of teratogenic or embryotoxic effects. These results are in agreement with those of other studies using somewhat different experimental plans.

Doses of 10 g/kg bw sodium cyclamate given to mice on day 5, 7 or 9 of pregnancy produced no significant increase in fetal mortality (Lorke, 1969b).

Multigeneration experiments, including studies on reproductive capacity and perinatal development, and teratological studies, performed with Swiss mice receiving 2 or 5% sodium cyclamate in the diet, revealed no pathological effects (Kroes et al., 1977).

Tanaka (1964) reported that sodium cyclamate is 40 times more toxic to fetal than to adult mice; however, these data appear to contradict all other results. Serious doubts have been raised about the data and experimental approach of Tanaka (Lorke, 1969b).

Taylor et al. (1968) performed an 11-month, three-generation study with rats using dietary levels of 1-3% sodium cyclamate. Although this study was complicated by an outbreak of infection and high mortality in all groups, data on mating, parturition and weaning gave no indication of an effect of sodium cyclamate on reproductive performance.

No indication of a primary embryotoxic effect was seen in female Wistar rats given 5% sodium cyclamate in their food for 20 days after mating (corresponding to 7.2 g cyclamate/kg bw ingested daily) (Luckhaus & Machemer, 1978).

The growth rate of offspring of rats given diets containing 10% calcium cyclamate was about 35% lower than that of controls with the same caloric intake. A decrease of about 15% was seen in the offspring of rats receiving 5% calcium cyclamate (Nees & Derse, 1965). With a reduced food intake (60% of normal), rats receiving 5% calcium cyclamate conceived, but the number of stillbirths was increased; rats that received 10% did not conceive (Nees & Derse, 1967).

It was reported in an abstract that in a three-generation reproduction study with Charles River CD rats, a dietary level of 5% calcium cyclamate led to decreased average weaning weights; animals maintained a low average bodyweight throughout the study (Taylor & Friedman, 1974).

No significant increase in fetal deaths, number of resorptions, decrease in survival from birth to weaning or teratogenic effects were seen in rats and hamsters treated with doses of calcium cyclamate corresponding to 50, 500 or 5000 mg/kg bw (Adkins et al., 1972).

The offspring of pregnant rats that were treated with 300 mg/l sodium and calcium cyclamate in drinking-water (equivalent to about 20 mg/kg bw daily) showed increased motor activity in behavioural tests; the effect persisted after discontinuation of cyclamate treatment (Stone et al., 1969a).

Fancher et al. (1968) found no significant toxicological changes in dogs treated with 0.5, 1.0 or 1.5 g/kg bw of a 10:1 combination of sodium cyclamate:sodium saccharin (the highest dose corresponding to 7.5 g per day in a 50-kg man) during pregnancy or in their offspring that received the same dose up to one year of age.

Oral administration of 500 or 2000 mg/kg bw sodium cyclamate to *Macaca mulatta* (rhesus) monkeys for different 4-day periods during the organogenesis stage (days 20-45 of pregnancy) had no adverse effect on the fetuses (Wilson, 1972).

Cyclohexylamine

Single i.p. injections of 61, 77 or 122 mg/kg bw cyclohexylamine given to Swiss-Webster mice on day 11 of pregnancy induced no teratogenic effects; however, only 41 fetuses at the high dose were evaluated. Increased fetolethality was noticed in litters treated with 77 or 122 mg/kg bw. Slight growth retardation was observed in the litters of all treated groups (Becker & Gibson, 1970; Gibson & Becker, 1971).

No substance-related teratogenic effects were observed in ICR mice treated orally with 20, 50 or 100 mg/kg bw cyclohexylamine either from day 0 to day 5 or from day 6 to day 11 of pregnancy. There was pronounced fetal growth retardation with the highest dose - which was lethal to some mothers - and a slight, but statistically significant growth retardation in other treated groups. The number of resorptions was increased in some treated groups, but was statistically significant only with the highest dose (Takano & Suzuki, 1971).

Male and female mice fed 0.11% cyclohexylamine sulphate in the diet (corresponding to about 136 mg cyclohexylamine/kg bw daily) were mated 10 weeks after beginning treatment. No effects were observed with respect to appearance, behaviour or weight; fertility was normal, and no biologically important increases in pre- and postimplantation losses were observed (Lorke & Machemer, 1975).

Multigeneration experiments, including studies on reproductive capacity and perinatal development, and teratological studies, performed with Swiss mice receiving 0.5% cyclohexylamine sulphate in the diet, showed a significant decrease in the number of implantation sites and in the number of liveborn fetuses as well as an increased perinatal mortality and a significant reduction in weight gain. No indication of a teratogenic effect was seen (Kroes et al., 1977).

^{14}C-Cyclohexylamine hydrochloride given to rhesus monkeys (10 mg/animal infused within 180 min) in the last trimester of pregnancy diffused across the placenta; maternal and fetal blood levels of radioactivity were virtually identical (Pitkin et al., 1969).

No substance-related teratogenic effects or effects on fetal growth or survival were seen in the fetuses of Wistar rats treated with 1.8-36 mg/kg bw cyclohexylamine or its sulphate on days 8-14 or 7-13 or pregnancy. The highest dose produced some symptoms of maternal toxicity (Omori et al., 1970; Tanaka et al., 1973).

No significant teratogenic or embryotoxic effects were found in rhesus monkeys treated with 25, 50 or 75 mg/kg bw cyclohexylamine for different 4-day periods during the phase of organogenesis (20-45 days of pregnancy) (Wilson, 1972).

Absorption, distribution, excretion and metabolism

^{14}C-Labelled sodium cyclamate (dose unspecified) had an average serum half-life of 8 hours in dogs and rats; 32% of the plasma cyclamate was not protein bound, and radioactivity was found in all tissues except brain. Milk levels of cyclamate in lactating dogs and rats administered calcium cyclamate were higher than blood levels and accounted for 0.001% of the dose/ml (Sonders & Wiegand, 1968; Ward & Zeman, 1971).

Sodium ^{14}C-cyclamate (100 mg/kg bw) was injected intravenously into two 21-day pregnant rats. After 5 min, the isotope was distributed relatively uniformly in maternal tissues, but the fetus contained little radioactivity. Seven hours later, however, a significant amount of the radioactivity was present in all fetal organs examined; most had disappeared from maternal organs (Schechter & Roth, 1971).

Sodium ^{14}C-cyclamate was given to two rhesus monkeys [4 mg/ animal] by continuous infusion (110 min) in the last trimester of pregnancy. Study of maternal-fetal transfer with the fetus *in utero* showed that the substance crossed the placenta. The maternal:fetal blood levels of radioactivity were about 4:1 at the end of infusion, suggesting a limited degree of transmission (Pitkin *et al.*, 1969).

Of ^{14}C-labelled cyclamate given orally to rats, 20-30% of the radioactivity was excreted in the urine, 70-80% in the faeces, and none in the expired air. Urinary excretion of radioactivity was higher in rats that could convert cyclamate to cyclohexylamine (WHO, 1971).

Oser *et al.* (1968) classified rats as either high, low or zero converters of cyclamate to cyclohexylamine. This conversion seems to be dose-related.

Cyclohexylamine has also been found in the urine of dogs, guinea-pigs, rabbits and monkeys following the administration of cyclamate (Asahina *et al.*, 1972; Golberg *et al.*, 1969; Ichibagase *et al.*, 1972; Parekh *et al.*, 1970).

In rhesus monkeys receiving 200 mg/kg bw cyclamate orally daily for several years, more than 99.5% was excreted unchanged. The principal metabolites found were cyclohexylamine, cyclohexanone and cyclohexanol (Coulston *et al.*, 1977).

Conversion in pigs, rats and rabbits increased with prolonged administration of cyclamates (Collings, 1971; Ichibagase *et al.*, 1972). The conversion is inhibited by neomycin and sulphaguanidine (Suenaga *et al.*, 1972).

Cyclamate is not metabolized by the liver, spleen or kidney tissue or blood of rats or rabbits fed cyclamate but is converted to cyclohexylamine when incubated anaerobically with the contents of caecum, colon or rectum or with faeces from cyclamate-pretreated rats or rabbits; *Clostridia* in rats and *Enterobacteria* in rabbits converted cyclamate to cyclohexylamine (Drasar *et al.*, 1972).

Rats fed diets containing 0.1% calcium cyclamate for 8 months then dosed with ^{14}C-cyclamate excreted traces of dicyclohexylamine, but no *N*-hydroxycyclohexylamine was detected (Prosky & O'Dell, 1971). Other authors have not detected dicyclohexylamine as a metabolite in rats (Sonders & Wiegand, 1968).

Cyclohexylamine is metabolized to a small extent (0.2%) to *N*-hydroxycyclohexyl-amine by rabbits (Elliott *et al.*, 1968). In the urine of rats, rabbits and guinea-pigs, other metabolites found in traces included cyclohexanol, cyclohexanone, *cis*- and *trans*-3- and 4-amino cyclohexanols and *trans*-cyclohexane-1,2-diol (Renwick & Williams, 1972a).

Mutagenicity and other short-term tests

The mutagenicity of cyclamates, cyclohexylamine and *N*-hydroxycyclohexylamine was reviewed by Cattanach (1976). Results of tests measuring the genetic activity of these substances indicate that both cyclamate and cyclohexylamine are clastogenic (cause chromosomal breaks); however, no mutagenic activity has been demonstrated in the limited number of mutagen assays for which results are available. There are no published data on testing in microbial and mammalian point mutation assays to date, except for a report in an abstract that *N*-hydroxycyclohexylamine, but not cyclohexylamine, increased the frequency of 8-azaguanine-resistant Chinese hamster cells *in vitro* (Chu & Bailiff, 1970).

Cyclohexylamine was negative in the *pol A* test for DNA repair-deficiency in *Escherichia coli* (Fluck *et al.*, 1976).

Chromosome damage occurred following treatment of onion root tips with a mixture of sodium cyclamate and saccharin (Sax & Sax, 1968). Chromosome breaks have been observed following treatment of human leucocytes with cyclamates *in vitro* (Ebenezer & Sadasivan, 1970; Lederer *et al.*, 1971; Perez Requejo, 1972; Stoltz *et al.*, 1970; Stone *et al.*, 1969b; Tokumitsu, 1971); similar activity has been reported for cyclohexylamine in kidney cells of kangaroo rats (Green *et al.*, 1970) and in human leucocytes (Stoltz *et al.*, 1970).

Cytogenetic effects were demonstrated *in vivo* in several tissues, including gonadal cells: Legator *et al.* (1969) detected an increased number of breaks in the spermatogonia of rats injected intraperitoneally with 10-50 mg/kg bw per day cyclohexylamine for 5 days. However, spermatogonia of hamsters given 5 oral doses of 2000 mg/kg bw sodium cyclamate (Machemer & Lorke, 1975) or 5 oral doses of 150 mg/kg bw cyclohexylamine sulphate (Machemer & Lorke, 1976) had no significant increases in chromosome aberrations; and calcium cyclamate did not increase the incidence of morphological sperm abnormalities in mice injected intraperitoneally with up to 500 mg/kg bw daily for 5 days (Wyrobek & Bruce, 1975). Chromosome damage was induced in bone-marrow cells of rats by i.p. administration of 10-50 mg/kg bw per day cyclohexylamine for 5 days (Legator *et al.*, 1969) and in those of gerbils similarly treated with 10-100 mg/kg bw calcium cyclamate for 5 days (Majumdar & Solomon, 1971a,b). Treatment of fetal lambs *in utero* with 50-250 mg/kg bw cyclohexylamine administered by catheter in the fetal jugular vein also caused chromosome damage in peripheral blood cells (Turner & Hutchinson, 1974).

Negative results have been obtained for cyclohexylamine and N-hydroxycyclohexyl-amine in the *Drosophila melanogaster* sex-linked recessive lethal test (Browning, 1972; Knaap *et al.*, 1973; Vogel & Chandler, 1974). No increase in recessive lethal mutations occurred following a 3-day treatment with 25 mM sodium cyclamate (Vogel & Chandler, 1974). Positive results in one experiment testing calcium cyclamate with this method were communicated in abstract form (Majumdar & Freedman, 1971).

Several tests for dominant lethal mutations in mice indicate that cyclohexylamine and its sulphate are not active in this system (Cattanach & Pollard, 1971; Epstein *et al.*, 1972; Lorke & Machemer, 1974). Petersen *et al.* (1972) recorded a significant increase in post-implantation losses in mice with 5 doses of 100 mg/kg bw cyclohexylamine; however, the validity of these results is questionable because the number of live implants in the triethylenemelamine-treated positive control group was larger than in the untreated control group. Tests for heritable translocations *in vivo* in mice were negative for both cyclohexylamine (Cattanach & Pollard, 1971) and sodium cyclamate (Leonard & Linden, 1972).

(b)   Humans

Toxic effects

Of 8 men taking 10 or 18 g sodium cyclamate per day for 3 months, 7 developed severe, persistent diarrhoea, and many had cyclohexylamine in the urine (Wills *et al.*, 1968). Continuous oral administration of 2-5 g sodium cyclamate per day for 3 years to patients with liver or kidney disease caused no obvious adverse clinical effects (Zöllner & Pieper, 1971; Zöllner & Schnelle, 1967).

Some skin conditions (e.g., pruritus, dermographia, urticaria, angioneurotic oedema) have been attributed to cyclamates (Feingold, 1968). A woman patient who took large amounts of calcium cyclamate had a photosensitive dermatitis and renal tubular acidosis associated with hypophosphataemia (Yong & Sanderson, 1969). Lamberg (1967) described a case of photosensitization in a black woman taking calcium cyclamate plus saccharin.

Teratogenic effects

Stone *et al.* (1971) studied 975 women delivered of children who were not mentally retarded and women delivered of 247 mentally retarded children. They found that more mothers of children with Down's syndrome and other causes of mental retardation had used artificial sweeteners before and during pregnancy than had controls (Table 4).

Table 4. Mothers of mentally retarded and normal children who had used artificial sweeteners during pregnancy

	Year of delivery		
	1959-61	1962-64	1965-69
Mothers of mentally retarded children	14/79 (17.7%)	26/115 (22.6%)	19/53 (35.8%)
Mothers of normal children	9/78 (11.5%) not significant	35/242 (14.5%) $\chi^2 = 4.75, P < 0.05$	141/655 (21.5%) $\chi^2 = 4.96, P < 0.05$
Relative risk[1]	1.7	1.7	2.0

In addition, the study showed that users of artificial sweeteners had an increased incidence of other adverse outcomes of pregnancy:'behavioural problems' (incidences-5.4%, 10/185, in children of artificial sweetener users and 2.0%, 16/790, in children of non-users) and 'physical anomalies' (mainly deformities of the bones and joints of the hip, leg and foot; incidences 4.8%, 9/185, in children of artificial sweetener users and 1.5%, 12/790, in children of non-users [P<0.01]) [Neither age, parity, smoking habits, the presence of diabetes mellitus nor socio-economic status were controlled for in the analysis, and no data were presented on how much artificial sweetener was used. The diverse effects found might argue against a direct effect of the artificial sweeteners, particularly in the absence of a prior expectation that exposure to such agents may cause such abnormalities. Further epidemiological data is needed before concluding that the use of artificial sweeteners in pregnancy is associated with fetal damage].

Absorption, distribution and excretion

When a dose of 100 mg sodium ^{14}C-cyclamate was injected intravenously to 5 women undergoing therapeutic abortion in early pregnancy, cyclamate crossed the placenta and was present in the fetal circulation at approximately one-quarter of maternal levels (maximum levels). It was widely distributed in fetal tissues, with the highest levels in liver, spleen and kidney (Pitkin *et al.*, 1970).

---

[1] Calculated by the Working Group

Metabolism

Kojima & Ichibagase (1966, 1969) found in several human subjects that up to 0.7% of an ingested dose of cyclamate was converted to cyclohexylamine, cyclohexanol, cyclo-hexanone and conjugated cyclohexanol, which were excreted in the urine. Enterococci in the intestine are probably the source of such conversion (Drasar *et al.*, 1972).

The metabolic conversion of cyclamate to cyclohexylamine has been studied in over 1000 human subjects. The urinary excretion of cyclohexylamine was found to vary from individual to individual and to fluctuate from day to day. About 10-30% of subjects converted cyclamate to cyclohexylamine: the majority of these converted <0.1-8% of ingested cyclamate; a few individuals converted up to 60%. Several studies indicate that the conversion of cyclamate to cyclohexylamine is inversely related to the dose of cyclamate (WHO, 1977). For more specific details, see Asahina *et al.* (1971), Collings (1971), Davis *et al.* (1969), Golberg *et al.* (1969), Leahy *et al.* (1967a,b), Litchfield & Swan (1971), Pawan (1970), Renwick & Williams (1972b), Sonders & Wiegand (1968), Williams (1971) and Wills *et al.* (1968).

Mutagenicity and other short-term tests

Chromosome breaks were observed in lymphocytes from human patients with chronic liver and kidney diseases who were dosed with 2-5 g per day cyclamates for 1-3 years. Sig-nificant differences were seen primarily between patients and controls, rather than between dosed and non-dosed patients (Bauchinger *et al.*, 1970).

Cyclohexylamine is a strong base and as such is irritating to the skin and mucous mem-branes and causes nausea and vomiting (Watrous & Schulz, 1950). It is a weak, indirect-acting sympathomimetic amine; doses of 10 mg/kg bw increase urinary excretion of catecholamines, but smaller doses cause increases in blood pressure (Eichelbaum *et al.*, 1974).

Cyclohexanol and *trans*-cyclohexane 1,2-diol were identified as metabolites of cyclo-hexylamine in human urine (Renwick & Williams, 1972a).

Dicyclohexylamine has not been detected as a metabolite of cyclamates in humans (Sonders & Wiegand, 1968).

3.3 Case reports and epidemiological studies

See **Studies in Humans of Cancer in Relation to the Consumption of Artificial, Non-nutritive Sweetening Agents**, pp. 171-183.

4. Summary of Data Reported and Evaluation

4.1 Experimental data

Sodium cyclamate has been tested by oral administration in two experiments in mice, one of which was a multigeneration study, and in three experiments in rats. A few benign and malignant bladder tumours were observed in rats, but the incidences were not statistically greater than those in controls in any single experiment. An increased incidence of lympho-sarcomas was seen in female but not in male mice in one experiment. Sodium cyclamate was also tested by oral administration in other experiments in mice, rats, hamsters and monkeys, but these experiments could not be evaluated because of various inadequacies or incomplete reporting.

Sodium cyclamate has also been tested in mice by bladder insertion (implantation) in one experiment: it increased the incidence of bladder carcinomas. When administered in one experiment by subcutaneous injection to rats, no tumours were seen at the site of injection.

Calcium cyclamate has been tested by oral administration in one two-generation experiment in rats; no difference in tumour incidence was seen between treated and control animals. Two further experiments in rats showing a few bladder tumours and one in hamsters were considered to be inadequate for evaluation. When administered by subcutaneous injection to rats, tumours were produced at the site of injection.

The combination of sodium cyclamate with sodium saccharin in a ratio of 10:1 has been tested by oral administration in a multigeneration experiment in mice and in two experiments in rats. In one study in rats, transitional-cell carcinomas in the bladder were produced in male animals given the highest dose; in the other study in rats and in the study in mice, there was no difference in tumour incidence between treated and control animals.

In one study in rats fed sodium cyclamate after receiving a single instillation into the bladder of a low dose of N-nitroso-N-methylurea, transitional-cell neoplasms of the bladder were produced. No such tumours were observed in animals that received N-nitroso-N-methyl-urea alone.

Cyclohexylamine has been tested by oral administration in two experiments in mice, one of which was a multigeneration study, and in four experiments in rats; there were no differences in tumour incidence between treated and control animals. A further experiment in rats was considered to be inadequate for evaluation.

The limited number of mutagenicity studies published give no evidence that cyclamates cause point mutations. Both cyclamates and cyclohexylamine cause chromosome damage.

There is no evidence that cyclamates and cyclohexylamine are teratogenic.

4.2 Human data

Mortality from bladder cancer has been investigated in two studies by examination of time trends in the United States and in England and Wales. These have shown no marked increase in incidence or mortality from bladder cancer following a substantial increase over a few years in the use of cyclamates and saccharin, but such studies are too insensitive to exclude completely a carcinogenic effect.

In two studies of cancer mortality in patients with diabetes mellitus (who, as a group, have been shown to consume larger quantities of artificial sweeteners than the general population), lower mortality from cancer at all sites was observed as compared with the general population; there was no excess of bladder cancer in particular. In a further study, the frequency of the mention of diabetes mellitus in death certificates of persons who had died of bladder cancers was compared with that in those of controls who had died of other cancers (excluding those of the lung and pancreas); in the presence of diabetes mellitus, there was no increase in the risk of bladder cancer. As there are differences other than artificial sweetener use between diabetics and the general population, such studies cannot exclude a small carcinogenic effect of these sweeteners.

Seven case-control studies were considered by the Working Group. Only two of these studies examined confounding factors in detail. Of these two, one suggested that use of nine or more tablets of artificial sweeteners per day was positively associated with risk for bladder cancer in men, but not in women, although in these small groups the results may have been due to chance, to unsuspected confounding factors, or to residual effects of those confounding factors that were considered in the analysis and could be shown to reduce the magnitude of the association. The other study that considered confounding factors suggested that there was no effect of the use of artificial sweeteners on the incidence of bladder cancer; the observed relative risk was 1.0 (indicating no increase in risk), but a relative risk below 1.4 could not be excluded. The other five case-control studies also showed no association, although they were limited by some inadequacies in experimental design.

In six of the seven case-control studies, women with bladder cancer showed a tendency to consume less artificial sweeteners than female controls. This observation suggests that there is no association between use of artificial sweeteners and bladder cancer in women.

4.3 Evaluation [1]

The experimental data provide *limited evidence* for the carcinogenicity of cyclamates in mice and rats. There is no conclusive evidence that cyclamates alone are carcinogenic when given by the oral route. There is evidence that they can promote the local action of a known carcinogen in the bladder. The available experimental data provide no evidence for the carcinogenicity of cyclohexylamine.

No adequate epidemiological data on cyclamates alone were available to the Working Group (see also saccharin, p. 156).

[1] See footnote pp. 182-183

5. References

Abbott Laboratories (1968) *Cyclohexylamine*, Bulletin 68-56, North Chicago, IL

Adkins, A., Hupp, E.W. & Gerdes, R.A. (1972) Biological activity of saccharins and cyclamates in golden hamsters (Abstract). *Texas J. Sci., 23,* 575

Althoff, J., Cardesa, A., Pour, P. & Shubik, P. (1975) A chronic study of artificial sweeteners in Syrian golden hamsters. *Cancer Lett., 1,* 21-24

American Conference of Governmental Industrial Hygienists (1978) TLVs[®] *Threshold Limit Values for Chemical Substances in Workroom Air Adopted by ACGIH for 1978,* Cincinnati, OH, p. 14

Anon. (1968) Chemical profiles: cyclohexylamine. *Chemical Marketing Reporter,* 1 July

Anon. (1977) Chemical profiles: cyclohexylamine. *Chemical Marketing Reporter,* 1 July

Asahina, M., Yamaka, T., Watanabe, K. & Sarrazin, G. (1971) Excretion of cyclohexylamine, a metabolite of cyclamate, in human urine. *Chem. pharm. Bull., 19,* 628-632

Asahina, M., Yamaka, T., Sarrazin, G. & Watanabe, K. (1972) Conversion of cyclamate to cyclohexylamine in guinea pig. *Chem. pharm. Bull., 20,* 102-108

Audrieth, L.F. & Sveda, M. (1944) Preparation and properties of some *N*-substituted sulfamic acids. *J. org. Chem., 9,* 89-101

Bailey, D.E., Morgareidge, K., Cox, G.E., Vogin, E.E. & Oser, B.L. (1972) Chronic toxicity, teratology, and mutagenicity studies with cyclohexylamine in rats (Abstract no. 148). *Toxicol. appl. Pharmacol., 22,* 330-331

Bajusz, E. (1969) Myocardial lesions: a reassessment of the toxicology of calcium cyclamate. *Nature, 223,* 406-407

Bauchinger, M., Schmid, E., Pieper, M. & Zöllner, N. (1970) Cytogenetic action of cyclamate on human peripheral lymphocytes *in vivo* (Ger.). *Dtsch. med. Wochensch., 95,* 2220-2223

Beck, K.M. (1969) *Sweeteners, nonnutritive.* In: Kirk, R.E. & Othmer, D.F., eds, *Encyclopedia of Chemical Technology,* 2nd ed., Vol. 19, New York, John Wiley & Sons, pp. 598-607

Becker, B.A. & Gibson, J.E. (1970)   Teratogenicity of cyclohexylamine in mammals. *Toxicol. appl. Pharmacol., 17,* 551-552

Berg, G.L., ed. (1979)   *Farm Chemicals Handbook 1979,* Willoughby, OH, Meister Publishing Co., p. D163

Bernier, J.-J., Bognel, J.-C. & Bognel, C. (1968)   Effects on the intestinal mucosa of the rat by prolonged administration of calcium cyclamate (Fr.). *Bull. Acad. natl Méd., 152,* 7-18

Brantom, P.G., Gaunt, I.F. & Grasso, P. (1973)   Long-term toxicity of sodium cyclamate in mice. *Food Cosmet. Toxicol., 11,* 735-746

Browning, L.S. (1972)   Failure to detect mutagenicity by injection of cyclohexylamine and *N'*-hydroxycyclohexylamine into *Drosophila* (Abstract no. 17). *EMS Newsl., 6,* 18-19

Bryan, G.T. & Ertürk, E. (1970)   Production of mouse urinary bladder carcinomas by sodium cyclamate. *Science, 167,* 996-998

Bundesminister der Justiz, ed. (1979)   *Bundesgesetzblatt,* 4. Anlage 2, Liste 12, Bonn, Bundesanzeiger Verlagsges. mbH, pp. 82-83

Carswell, T.S. & Morrill, H.L. (1937)   Cyclohexylamine and dicyclohexylamine. *Ind. Eng. Chem., 29,* 1247-1251

Cattanach, B.M. (1976)   The mutagenicity of cyclamates and their metabolites. *Mutat. Res., 39,* 1-28

Cattanach, B.M. & Pollard, C.E. (1971)   Mutagenicity tests with cyclohexylamine in the mouse. *Mutat. Res., 12,* 472-474

Chu, E.Y.H. & Bailiff, E.G. (1970)   Mutagenicity test of the metabolic derivatives of cyclamates in mammalian cell cultures (Abstract no. 28). *EMS Newsl., 3,* 39

Classen, H.G., Marquardt, P. & Späth, M. (1968)   Sympathicomimetic effects of cyclohexylamine (Ger). *Arzneimittel-Forsch., 18,* 590-594

Collings, A.J. (1971)   *Metabolism of sodium cyclamate.* In: Birch, G.G., ed., *Sweetness Sweeteners,* London, Applied Science Publishers Ltd, pp. 51-68

Coulston, F., McChesney, E.W. & Golberg, L. (1975)   Long-term administration of artificial sweeteners to the rhesus monkey *(M. mulatta). Food Cosmet. Toxicol., 13,* 297-299

Coulston, F., McChesney, E.W. & Benitz, K.-F. (1977) Eight-year study of cyclamate in rhesus monkeys (Abstract no. 80). *Toxicol. appl. Pharmacol., 41,* 164-165

Davis, T.R.A., Adler, N. & Opsahl, J.C. (1969) Excretion of cyclohexylamine in subjects ingesting sodium cyclamate. *Toxicol. appl. Pharmacol., 15,* 106-116

Drasar, B.S., Renwick, A.G. & Williams, R.T. (1972) The role of the gut flora in the metabolism of cyclamate. *Biochem. J., 129,* 881-890

Ebenezer, L.N. & Sadasivan, G. (1970) *In vitro* effect of cyclamates on human chromosomes. *Q. J. surg. Sci., 6,* 116-118

Eichelbaum, M., Hengstmann, J.H., Rost, H.D., Brecht, T. & Dengler, H.J. (1974) Pharmacokinetics, cardiovascular and metabolic actions of cyclohexylamine in man. *Arch. Toxikol., 31,* 243-263

Elliott, T.H., Lee-Yoong, N.Y. & Tao, R.C.C. (1968) The metabolism of cyclohexylamine in rabbits. *Biochem. J., 109,* 11P-12P

Epstein, S.S., Arnold, E., Andrea, J., Bass, W. & Bishop, Y. (1972) Detection of chemical mutagens by the dominant lethal assay in the mouse. *Toxicol. appl. Pharmacol., 23,* 288-325

Ershoff, B.H. (1976) Protective effects of cholestyramine in rats fed a low-fiber diet containing toxic doses of sodium cyclamate or amaranth. *Proc. Soc. exp. Biol. (N.Y.), 152,* 253-256

Ershoff, B.H. (1977) Effects of dietary carbohydrate on sodium cyclamate toxicity in rats fed a purified, low-fiber diet. *Proc. Soc. exp. Biol. (N.Y.), 154,* 65-68

Ershoff, B.H. & Bajwa, G.S. (1974) Inhibitory effect of sodium cyclamate and sodium saccharin on tumor induction by 2-acetylaminofluorene in rats. *Proc. Soc. exp. Biol. (N.Y.), 145,* 1293-1297

Erskine, J.W. & Williams, A.F. (1970) Determination of dicyclohexylamine in sodium cyclamate. *Talanta, 17,* 244-246 [*Chem. Abstr., 72,* 117457g]

Fancher, O.E., Palazzolo, R.J., Blockhus, L., Weinberg, M.S. & Calandra, J.C. (1968) Chronic studies with sodium saccharin and sodium cyclamate in dogs (Abstract no. 15). *Toxicol. appl. Pharmacol., 12,* 291

Feingold, B.F. (1968) Recognition of food additives as a cause of symptoms of allergy. *Ann. Allergy, 26,* 309-313

Fitzhugh, O.G., Nelson, A.A. & Frawley, J.P. (1951) A comparison of the chronic toxicities of synthetic sweetening agents. *J. Am. pharm. Assoc., 40,* 583-586

Fluck, E.R., Poirier, L.A. & Ruelius, H.W. (1976) Evaluation of a DNA polymerase-deficient mutant of *E. coli* for the rapid detection of carcinogens. *Chem. -biol. Interactions, 15,* 219-231

Friedman, L., Richardson, H.L., Richardson, M.E., Lethco, E.J., Wallace, W.C. & Sauro, F.M. (1972) Toxic response of rats to cyclamates in chow and semisynthetic diets. *J. natl Cancer Inst., 49,* 751-764

Fritz, H. & Hess, R. (1968) Prenatal development in the rat following the administration of cyclamate, saccharin and sucrose. *Experientia, 24,* 1140-1141

Furuya, T., Kawamata, K., Kaneko, T., Uchida, O., Horiuchi, S. & Ikeda, Y. (1975) Long-term toxicity study of sodium cyclamate and saccharin sodium in rats (Abstract). *Jpn. J. Pharmacol., 25,* 55P-56P

Gaunt, I.F., Sharratt, M., Grasso, P., Lansdown, A.B.G. & Gangolli, S.D. (1974) Short-term toxicity of cyclohexylamine hydrochloride in the rat. *Food Cosmet. Toxicol., 12,* 609-624

Gaunt, I.F., Hardy, J., Grasso, P., Gangolli, S.D. & Butterworth, K.R. (1976) Long-term toxicity of cyclohexylamine hydrochloride in the rat. *Food Cosmet. Toxicol., 14,* 255-267

Gibson, J.E. & Becker, B.A. (1971) Teratogenicity of structural truncates of cyclophosphamide in mice. *Teratology, 4,* 141-150

Golberg, L., Parekh, C., Patti, A. & Soike, K. (1969) Cyclamate degradation in mammals and *in vitro* (Abstract no. 107). *Toxicol. appl. Pharmacol., 14,* 654

Göttinger, E., Hagmüller, K., Hellauer, H. & Vinazzer, H. (1968) On the effect of the sweetening agent cyclamate on the liver parenchyma, the corresponding enzymes and the coagulation factors of the blood (Ger.). *Wien. klin. Wschr., 80,* 328-332

Grasso, P., Gangolli, S.D., Golberg, L. & Hooson, J. (1971) Physicochemical and other factors determining local sarcoma production by food additives. *Food Cosmet. Toxicol., 9,* 463-478

Green, S., Palmer, K.A. & Legator, M.S. (1970) *In vitro* cytogenetic investigation of calcium cyclamate, cyclohexylamine and triflupromazine. *Food Cosmet. Toxicol., 8,* 617-623

Guven, K.C. & Savaskan, F. (1974) Identification of saccharin and cyclamate by thin-layer chromatography (Turk.). *Eczacilik Bul., 16,* 60-64 [*Chem. Abstr., 82,* 103240a]

Hagmüller, K., Hellauer, H., Winkler, R. & Zangger, J. (1969) New histological findings and further experimental data on the question of cyclamate tolerance in guinea-pigs (Ger.). *Wien. klin. Wschr., 81,* 927-938

Hampton, C.M. & Myers, R.L. (1976) Effects of cyclamate calcium on the immune response in rabbits. *Arch. environ. Health, 31,* 47-49, 51-53

Hancock, E.G., ed. (1975) *Benzene and its Industrial Derivatives,* New York, Halstead Press, pp. 234, 500-501

Hardy, J., Gaunt, I.F., Hooson, J., Hendy, R.J. & Butterworth, K.R. (1976) Long-term toxicity of cyclohexylamine hydrochloride in mice. *Food Cosmet. Toxicol., 14,* 269-276

Hicks, R.M. & Chowaniec, J. (1977) The importance of synergy between weak carcinogens in the induction of bladder cancer in experimental animals and humans. *Cancer Res., 37,* 2943-2949

Hicks, R.M., Chowaniec, J. & Wakefield, J.St.J. (1978) *Experimental induction of bladder tumors by a two-stage system.* In: Slaga, T.J., Sivak, A. & Boutwell, R.K., eds, *Carcinogenesis,* Vol. 2, *Mechanisms of Tumor Promotion and Cocarcinogenesis,* New York, Raven Press, pp. 475-489

Homburger, F. (1978) *Negative lifetime carcinogen studies in rats and mice fed 50,000 ppm saccharin.* In: Galli, C.L., Pasletti, R. & Vettorazzi, G., eds, *Chemical Toxicology of Food,* Amsterdam, Elsevier/North Holland Biomedical Press, pp. 359-373

Howard, J.W., Fazio, T., Klimeck, B.A. & White, R.H. (1969a) Determination of cyclohexylamine in various artificially sweetened foods and artificial sweeteners. *J. Assoc. off. anal. Chem., 52,* 492-500

Howard, J.W., Fazio, T., Williams, B.K. & White, R.H. (1969b) Determination of dicyclohexylamine in cyclamates. *J. Assoc. off. anal. Chem., 52,* 1195-1199

Hwang, K. (1966) Mechanism of the laxative effect of sodium sulfate, sodium cyclamate and calcium cyclamate. *Arch. int. Pharmacodyn., 163,* 302-340

IARC (1979) *Information Bulletin on the Survey of Chemicals Being Tested for Carcinogenicity, No. 8,* Lyon, p. 387

Ichibagase, H., Kojima, S., Suenaga, A. & Inoue, K. (1972) Studies on synthetic sweetening agents. XVI. Metabolism of sodium cyclamate. 5. The metabolism of sodium cyclamate in rabbits and rats after prolonged administration of sodium cyclamate. *Chem. pharm. Bull., 20,* 1093-1101

International Labour Organisation (1971) *Encyclopedia of Occupational Safety and Health,* Vol. 1, Geneva, International Labour Office, p. 92

Ivashchenko, L.N., Zosim, Z.L. & Beilis, J. (1975) Polarographic determination of amines inhibiting atmospheric corrosion of metals (Russ.). *Sb. Tr. Ukr. Nauchno-Issled. Inst. Tsellyul. -Bum. Prom-sti., 18,* 125-129 [*Chem. Abstr., 88,* 202617j]

Klotzsche, C. (1969) On the teratogenic and embryotoxic effect of cyclamate, saccharin and sucrose (Ger.). *Arzneimittel-Forsch., 19,* 925-928

Knaap, A.G.A.C., Kramers, P.G.N. & Sobels, F.H. (1973) Lack of mutagenicity of the cyclamate metabolites in *Drosophila. Mutat. Res., 21,* 341-344

Kojima, S. & Ichibagase, H. (1966) Studies on synthetic sweetening agents. VIII. Cyclohexylamine, a metabolite of sodium cyclamate. *Chem. pharm. Bull., 14,* 971-974

Kojima, S. & Ichibagase, H. (1969) Studies on synthetic sweetening agents. XIV. Metabolism of sodium cyclamate. 3. On metabolites of sodium cyclamate in human. *Chem. pharm. Bull., 17,* 2620-2625

Kroes, R., Peters, P.W.J., Berkvens, J.M., Verschuuren, H.G., De Vries, T. & van Esch, G.J. (1977) Long-term toxicity and reproduction study (including a teratogenicity study) with cyclamate, saccharin and cyclohexylamine. *Toxicology, 8,* 285-300

Lamberg, S.I. (1967) A new photosensitizer. The artificial sweetener cyclamate. *J. Am. med. Assoc., 201,* 747-750 (121-124)

La Rotonda, M.I. & Ferrara, L. (1975) Detection and determination of synthetic sweeteners in foods and pharmaceutical preparations (Ital.). *Boll. Soc. Ital. Biol. sper., 51,* 690-695 [*Chem. Abstr., 84,* 98929s]

Leahy, J.S., Wakefield, M. & Taylor, T. (1967a) Urinary excretion of cyclohexylamine following oral administration of sodium cyclamate to man. *Food Cosmet. Toxicol., 5,* 447

Leahy, J.S., Taylor, T. & Rudd, C.J. (1967b) Cyclohexylamine excretors among human volunteers given cyclamate. *Food Cosmet. Toxicol., 5,* 595-596

Lederer, J., Collin, J.-P., Pottier-Arnould, A.-M. & Gondry, E. (1971) The cytogenetic and teratogenic effect of cyclamate and its metabolites (Fr.). *Thérapeutique, 47,* 357-363

Legator, M.S., Palmer, K.A., Green, S. & Peterson, K.W. (1969) Cytogenetic studies in rats of cyclohexylamine, a metabolite of cyclamate. *Science, 165,* 1139-1140

Leonard, A. & Linden, G. (1972) Observations on the mutagenic properties of cyclamates in mammals (Fr.). *C.R. Soc. Biol. (Paris), 166,* 468-470

Litchfield, M.H. & Swan, A.A.B. (1971) Cyclohexylamine production and physiological measurements in subjects ingesting sodium cyclamate. *Toxicol. appl. Pharmacol., 18,* 535-541

Lorke, D. (1969a) Studies on the embryotoxic and teratogenic effects of cyclamate and saccharin in the mouse (Ger.). *Arzneimittel-Forsch., 19,* 920-922

Lorke, D. (1969b) Toxicity of cyclamate on the mouse embryo (Ger.). *Arzneimittel-Forsch., 19,* 923-925

Lorke, D. & Machemer, L. (1974) Investigation of cyclohexylamine sulfate for dominant lethal effects in the mouse. *Toxicology, 2,* 231-237

Lorke, D. & Machemer, L. (1975) The effect of several weeks' treatment of male and female mice with saccharin, cyclamate or cyclohexylamine sulphate on fertility and dominant lethal effects (Ger.). *Humangenetik, 26,* 199-205

Löser, E. (1977) Subchronic toxicological studies with sodium cyclamate in dogs (Ger.). *Arzneimittel-Forsch., 27,* 128-131

Luckhaus, G. & Machemer, L. (1978) Histological examination of perinatal eye development in the rat after ingestion of sodium cyclamate and sodium saccharin during pregnancy. *Food Cosmet. Toxicol., 16,* 7-11

Machemer, L. & Lorke, D. (1975) Method for testing mutagenic effects of chemicals on spermatogonia of the Chinese hamster. Results obtained with cyclophosphamide, saccharin and cyclamate. *Arzneimittel-Forsch., 25,* 1889-1896

Machemer, L. & Lorke, D. (1976) Evaluation of the mutagenic potential of cyclohexylamine on spermatogonia of the Chinese hamster. *Mutat. Res., 40,* 243-250

Majumdar, S.K. & Freedman, C. (1971) Mutation test of calcium cyclamate in *Drosophila melanogaster* (Abstract). *Drosophila Inf. Serv., 46,* 114

Majumdar, S.K. & Solomon, M. (1971a) Chromosome changes in Mongolian gerbil following calcium cyclamate administration. *Nucleus, 14,* 168-170

Majumdar, S.K. & Solomon, M. (1971b) Cytogenetic studies of calcium cyclamate in *Meriones unguiculatus* (gerbil) *in vivo. Can. J. Genet. Cytol., 13,* 189-194

Marhold, J., Hub, M., Ruffer, F. & Andrysová, O. (1967) On the carcinogenicity of dicyclo-hexylamine. *Neoplasma, 14,* 177-180

Mason, P.L. & Thompson, G.R. (1977) Testicular effects of cyclohexylamine hydro-chloride in the rat. *Toxicology, 8,* 143-156

Matsumura, R. & Kohei, H. (1976) Studies on the formation of cyclohexylamine and N-methylcyclohexylamine from bromhexine in animals and man, and simultaneous determination of cyclohexylamine and N-methylcyclohexylamine by gas chroma-tography. *J. Chromatogr., 117,* 383-391

Miyata, T., Kase, Y., Kamikawa, Y., Kataoka, M., Kikuchi, K. & Touchi, T. (1969) Pharmacological characteristics of cyclohexylamine, one of metabolites of cyclamate. *Life Sci., 8,* 843-853

Mohr, U., Green, U., Althoff, J. & Schneider, P. (1978) *Syncarcinogenic action of saccha-rin and sodium-cyclamate in the induction of bladder tumours in MNU-pretreated rats.* In: Guggenheim, B., ed., *Health and Sugar Substitutes,* Basel, Karger, pp. 64-69

Nagasawa, K., Shinozuka, T. & Ogamo, A. (1974) Gas chromatographic determination of microamounts of cyclamate by trifluoroacetolysis (Jpn.). *Eisei Kagaku, 20,* 337-340 [*Chem. Abstr., 83,* 22049p]

Nasierowska, Z. (1975) Research and determination of artificial sweetening materials in some pharmaceutical preparations. I. Isolation and identification of saccharin, sodium saccharin, sodium cyclamate and dulcin with thin-layer chromatography (Pol.). *Farm. Pol., 31,* 940-945 [*Chem. Abstr.., 84,* 111753b]

Nathan, C.C. (1965) *Corrosion inhibitors.* In: Kirk, R.E. & Othmer, D.F., eds, *Encyclo-pedia of Chemical Technology,* 2nd ed., Vol. 6, New York, John Wiley & Sons, pp. 330-332

National Formulary Board (1970) *National Formulary XIII,* 13th ed., Washington DC, American Pharmaceutical Association, pp. 118-121, 642-645

Nees, P.O. & Derse, P.H. (1965) Feeding and reproduction of rats fed calcium cyclamate. *Nature, 208,* 81-82

Nees, P.O. & Derse, P.H. (1967) Effect of feeding calcium cyclamate to rats. *Nature, 211,* 1191-1195

Omori, Y., Kuwamura, T., Tanaka, S. & Nakaura, S. (1970) Experimental studies on cyclohexylamine in relation to congenital anomalies. *EMS Newsl., 3,* 30

Oser, B.L., Carson, S., Vogin, E.E. & Sonders, R.C. (1968) Conversion of cyclamate to cyclohexylamine in rats. *Nature, 220,* 178-179

Oser, B.L., Carson, S., Cox, G.E., Vogin, E.E. & Sternberg, S.S. (1975) Chronic toxicity study of cyclamate:saccharin (10:1) in rats. *Toxicology, 4,* 315-330

Oser, B.L., Carson, S., Cox, G.E., Vogin, E.E. & Sternberg, S.S. (1976) Long-term and multigeneration toxicity studies with cyclohexylamine hydrochloride. *Toxicology, 6,* 47-65

Parekh, C., Goldberg, E.K. & Goldberg, L. (1970) Fate of sodium cyclamate-^{14}C in the rhesus monkey (*M. mulatta*) (Abstract no. 26). *Toxicol. appl. Pharmacol., 17,* 282

Pawan, G.L.S. (1970) Dietary cyclamate and cyclohexylamine excretion in man (Abstract). *Proc. Nutr. Soc., 29,* 10A-11A

Perez Requejo, J.L. (1972) *In vitro* effect of sodium cyclamate on human chromosomes (Sp.). *Sangre, 17,* 386-394

Petersen, K.W., Legator, M.S. & Figge, F.H. (1972) Dominant-lethal effects of cyclohexylamine in C57B1/Fe mice. *Mutat. Res., 14,* 126-129

Pitkin, R.M., Reynolds, W.A. & Filer, L.J. (1969) Cyclamate and cyclohexylamine: transfer across the hemocharial placenta. *Proc. Soc. exp. Biol. (N.Y.), 132,* 993-995

Pitkin, R.M., Reynolds, W.A. & Filer, L.J., Jr (1970) Placental transmission and fetal distribution of cyclamate in early human pregnancy. *Am. J. Obstet. Gynecol., 108,* 1043-1050

Pliss, G.B. (1958) The carcinogenic activity of dicyclohexylamine and its nitrite salt. *Vopr. Onkol., 3,* 659-668

Price, J.M., Biava, C.G., Oser, B.L., Vogin, E.E., Steinfeld, J. & Ley, H.L. (1970) Bladder tumors in rats fed cyclohexylamine or high doses of a mixture of cyclamate and saccharin. *Science, 167,* 1131-1132

Prosky, L. & O'Dell, R.G. (1971) *In vivo* conversion of ^{14}C-labeled cyclamate to cyclohexylamine. *J. pharm. Sci., 60,* 1341-1343

Rainey, W.T., Christie, W.H. & Lijinsky, W. (1978) Mass spectrometry of *N*-nitrosamines. *Biomed. Mass Spectrom., 5,* 395-408

Renwick, A.G. & Williams, R.T. (1972a) The metabolites of cyclohexylamine in man and certain animals. *Biochem. J., 129,* 857-867

Renwick, A.G. & Williams, R.T. (1972b) The fate of cyclamate in man and other species. *Biochem. J., 129,* 869-879

Richards, R.K., Taylor, J.D., O'Brien, J.L. & Duescher, H.O. (1951) Studies on cyclamate sodium (Sucaryl sodium), a new noncaloric sweetening agent. *J. Am. pharm. Assoc., 40,* 1-6

Richardson, H.L., Richardson, M.E., Stewart, H.L., Lethco, E.J. & Wallace, W.C. (1972) Urinary bladder carcinoma and other pathological alterations in rats fed cyclamates (Abstract no. 6). *Proc. Am. Assoc. Cancer Res., 13,* 2

Roe, F.J.C., Levy, L.S. & Carter, R.L. (1970) Feeding studies on sodium cyclamate, saccharin and sucrose for carcinogenic and tumour-promoting activity. *Food Cosmet. Toxicol., 8,* 135-145

Rudali, G., Coezy, E. & Muranyi-Kovacs, I. (1969) Studies on the carcinogenic effect of sodium cyclamate in mice (Fr.). *C.R. Acad. Sci (Paris), 269,* 1910-1912

Sandridge, R.L. & Staley, H.B. (1978) *Amines by reduction.* In: Kirk, R.E. & Othmer, D.F., eds, *Encyclopedia of Chemical Technology,* 3rd ed., Vol. 2, New York, John Wiley & Sons, pp. 313, 360

Sax, K. & Sax, H.J. (1968) Possible mutagenic hazards of some food additives, beverages and insecticides. *Jpn. J. Genet., 43,* 89-94

Schechter, P.J. & Roth, L.J (1971) Whole-body autoradiography of ^{14}C sodium cyclamate in pregnant and fetal rats. *Toxicol. appl. Pharmacol., 20,* 130-133

Schmähl, D. (1973) Lack of a carcinogenic effect of cyclamate, cyclohexylamine and saccharin in rats (Ger.). *Arzneimittel-Forsch., 23,* 1466-1470

Schmähl, D. & Krüger, F.W. (1972) Lack of a syncarcinogenic effect of cyclamate on the occurrence of bladder cancer with butyl-butanol-nitrosamine in rats (Ger.). *Arzneimittel-Forsch., 22,* 999-1000

Shimada, K., Matsumoto, U., Hirago, T., Shibusawa, Y. & Nagase, Y. (1977) Determination of sodium cyclamate by isotope dilution analysis (Jpn.). *Yakugaku Zasshi, 97,* 849-854 [*Chem. Abstr., 87,* 199241d]

Sieber, S.M. & Adamson, R.H. (1978) *Long-term studies on the potential carcino-genicity of artificial sweeteners in non-human primates.* In: Guggenheim, B., ed., *Health and Sugar Substitutes,* Basel, Karger, pp. 266-271

The Society of Dyers and Colourists (1971) *Colour Index,* 3rd ed., Vol. 4, Bradford, Yorkshire, UK, p. 4759

Sonders, R.C. & Wiegand, R.G. (1968) Absorption and excretion of cyclamate in animals and man (Abstract no. 16). *Toxicol. appl. Pharmacol., 12,* 291

Stein, A.A., Serrone, D.M. & Coulston, F. (1967) Ultrastructural and biochemical studies of sodium cyclamate (Abstract no. 9). *Toxicol. appl. Pharmacol., 10,* 381

Stoltz, D.R., Khera, K.S., Bendall, R. & Gunner, S.W. (1970) Cytogenetic studies with cyclamate and related compounds. *Science, 167,* 1501-1502

Stone, D., Matalka, E. & Riordan, J. (1969a) Hyperactivity in rats bred and raised on relatively low amounts of cyclamates. *Nature, 224,* 1326-1328

Stone, D., Lamson, E., Chang, Y.S. & Pickering, K.W. (1969b) Cytogenetic effects of cyclamates on human cells *in vitro. Science, 164,* 568-569

Stone, D., Matalka, E. & Pulaski, B. (1971) Do artificial sweeteners ingested in pregnancy affect the offspring? *Nature, 231,* 53

Suenaga, A., Kojima, S. & Ichibagase, H. (1972) Studies on synthetic sweetening agents. XVII. Metabolism of sodium cyclamate. 6. Influences of neomycin and sulfaguani-dine on metabolism of sodium cyclamate. *Chem. pharm. Bull., 20,* 1357-1361

Takano, K. & Suzuki, M. (1971) Cyclohexylamine, a chromosome-aberration inducing substance: no teratogenicity in mice (Jpn.). *Congenital Anomalies, 11,* 51-57

Tanaka, R. (1964) LD$_{50}$ of the saccharin or cyclamate for mice embryo in the 7th day of pregnancy (fetal median lethal dose: FLD$_{50}$). *J. Iwate med. Assoc., 16,* 330-337

Tanaka, S., Nakaura, S., Kawashima, K., Nagao, S., Kuwamura, T. & Omori, Y. (1973) Studies on the teratogenicity of food additives. 2. Effects of cyclohexylamine and cyclohexylamine sulfate on the fetal development in rats. *J. Food Hyg. Soc., 14,* 542-548

Taylor, J.D., Richards, R.K., Wiegand, R.G. & Weinberg, M.S. (1968) Toxicological studies with sodium cyclamate and saccharin. *Food Cosmet. Toxicol., 6,* 313-327

Taylor, J.M. & Friedman, L. (1974) Combined chronic feeding and three-generation reproduction study of sodium saccharin in the rat (Abstract no. 200). *Toxicol. appl. Pharmacol., 29,* 154

Tokumitsu, T. (1971) Some aspects of cytogenetic effects of sodium cyclamate on human leucocytes *in vitro. Proc. Jpn Acad., 47,* 635-639

Toth, B. (1972) A toxicity method with calcium cyclamate for chronic carcinogenesis experiments. *Tumori, 58,* 137-141

Turner, J.H. & Hutchinson, D.L. (1974) Cyclohexylamine mutagenicity: an *in vivo* evaluation utilizing fetal lambs. *Mutat. Res., 26,* 407-412

US Food & Drug Administration (1969a) Exemption of certain food additives from the requirement of tolerances. Cyclamic acid and its salts. *Fed. Regist., 34,* 17063-17064

US Food & Drug Administration (1969b) Abbreviated new-drug applications for cyclamates. *Fed. Regist., 34,* 20426-20427

US Food & Drug Administration (1970) Revocations regarding cyclamate-containing products intended for drug use. *Fed. Regist., 35,* 13644-13645

US Food & Drug Administration (1978) Food and drugs. *US Code Fed. Regul.,* Title 21, part 173.310, pp. 473-474

US International Trade Commission (1977) *Synthetic Organic Chemicals, US Production and Sales, 1976,* USITC Publication 833, Washington DC, US Government Printing Office, pp. 37, 52, 193

US International Trade Commission (1978a) *Synthetic Organic Chemicals, US Production and Sales, 1977,* USITC Publication 920, Washington DC, US Government Printing Office, pp. 47, 61, 64, 200

US International Trade Commission (1978b) *Imports of Benzenoid Chemicals and Products, 1977,* USITC Publication 900, Washington DC, US Government Printing Office, pp. 16, 18

US Tariff Commission (1951) *Synthetic Organic Chemicals, US Production and Sales, 1950,* Report No. 173, Second Series, Washington DC, US Government Printing Office, p. 108

US Tariff Commission (1954) *Synthetic Organic Chemicals, US Production and Sales, 1953,* Report No. 194, Second Series, Washington DC, US Government Printing Office, p. 114

US Tariff Commission (1969) *Synthetic Organic Chemicals, US Production and Sales, 1967,* TC Publication 295, Washington DC, US Government Printing Office, p. 12

US Tariff Commission (1970) *Imports of Benzenoid Chemicals and Products, 1969,* TC Publication 328, Washington DC, US Government Printing Office, p. 12

Vogel, E. & Chandler, J.L.R. (1974) Mutagenicity testing of cyclamate and some pesticides in *Drosophila melanogaster. Experientia, 30,* 621-623

Wade, A., ed. (1977) *Martindale, The Extra Pharmacopoeia,* 27th ed., London, The Pharmaceutical Press, pp. 611, 614-615

Ward, V.L. & Zeman, F.J. (1971) Distribution of ^{14}C-cyclamate in the lactating rat. *J. Nutr., 101,* 1635-1646

Watrous, R.M. & Schulz, H.N. (1950) Cyclohexylamine, *p*-chlornitrobenzene, 2-amino-pyridine: toxic effects in industrial use. *Ind. Med. Surg., 19,* 317-320

WHO (1967) Toxicological evaluation of some flavouring substances and non-nutritive sweetening agents. *WHO/Food Add./68.33,* pp. 82-99

WHO (1971) Toxicological evaluation of some extraction solvents and certain other substances. *WHO/Food Add./70.39,* pp. 12-31

WHO (1977) Summary of toxicological data of certain food additives. *WHO Food Add. Ser., No. 12,* pp. 116-123

Wiegand, R.G. (1978) *Practical considerations for synthetic sweeteners: past, present and future - cyclamates.* In: Shaw, J.H. & Roussos, G.G., eds, *Sweeteners and Dental Caries,* Arlington, VA, Information Retrieval, Inc., pp. 263-267

Williams, R.T. (1971) The metabolism of certain drugs and food chemicals in man. *Ann. N.Y. Acad. Sci., 179,* 141-154

Wills, J.H., Jameson, E., Stoewsand, G. & Coulston, F. (1968) A three-month study of daily intake of sodium cyclamate by man (Abstract no. 17). *Toxicol. appl. Pharmacol., 12,* 292

Wilson, J.G. (1972) *Use of primates in teratological investigations.* In: Goldsmith, E.I. & Moor-Jankowski, J., eds, *Medical Primatology,* Basel, Karger, pp. 286-295

Windholz, M., ed. (1976) *The Merck Index,* 9th ed., Rahway, NJ, Merck & Co., pp. 352, 357

Wyrobek, A.J. & Bruce, W.R. (1975) Chemical induction of sperm abnormalities in mice. *Proc. natl Acad. Sci. (USA), 72,* 4425-4429

Yamamura, H.I., Lee, I.P. & Dixon, R.L. (1968) Study of the sympathomimetic action of cyclohexylamine, a possible metabolite of cyclamate. *J. pharm. Sci., 57,* 1132-1134

Yong, J.M. & Sanderson, K.V. (1969) Photosensitive dermatitis and renal tubular acidosis after ingestion of calcium cyclamate. *Lancet, ii,* 1273-1275

Zöllner, N. & Pieper, M. (1971) Results of a three-year clinical study with cyclamate (Ger.). *Arzneimittel-Forsch., 21,* 431-432

Zöllner, N. & Schnelle, K. (1967) Clinical studies on the toxicity of long-term administration of cyclamate to patients with liver and kidney diseases (Ger.). *Arzneimittel-Forsch., 17,* 1568-1573

(SACCHARIN, SODIUM SACCHARIN, CALCIUM SACCHARIN
& *ortho*-TOLUENESULPHONAMIDE)

1. Chemical and Physical Data

Saccharin[1]

1.1 Synonyms and trade names

Chem. Abstr. Services Reg. No.: 81-07-2

Chem. Abstr. Name: 1,2-Benzisothiazol-3(2*H*)-one,1,1-dioxide

Synonyms: Anhydro-*ortho*-sulphaminebenzoic acid; 1,2-benzisothiazolinone, 1,1-dioxide; 1,2-benzisothiazolin-3-one, 1,1-dioxide; 3-benzisothiazolinone 1,1-dioxide; benzoic sulphimide; *ortho*-benzoic sulphimide; benzoic sulphinide; benzosulphimide; benzo-2-sulphimide; *ortho*-benzosulphimide; benzo-sulphinide; *ortho*-benzoyl sulphimide; 1,2-dihydro-2-ketobenzisosulphonazole; 2,3-dihydro-3-oxobenzisosulphon-azole; 3-hydroxybenzisothiazole-*S,S*-dioxide; insoluble saccharin; saccharimide; saccharin acid; saccharine; saccharin insoluble; *ortho*-sulphobenzimide; *ortho*-sulpho-benzoic acid imide; 2-sulphobenzoic imide

Trade names: Assugrin vollsuss (also contains sodium cyclamate); Garantose; Glucid; Gluside; Hermesetas; Kandiset; Natreen (also contains sodium cyclamate); Sacarina; 550 Saccharin; Saccharina; Saccharinol; Saccharinose; Saccharol; Saxin; Sucre Edulcor; Sucrette; Sykose; Zaharina

1.2 Structural and molecular formulae and molecular weight

$C_7H_5NO_3S$ Mol. wt: 183.2

---

[1] The name 'saccharin' is sometimes (e.g., in government regulations) applied to the ammonium, calcium and sodium salts as well as to the free acid.

1.3 Chemical and physical properties of the pure substance

From Wade (1977) and Windholz (1976), unless otherwise specified

(a) *Description:* White crystalline powder with an intensely sweet taste

(b) *Melting-point:* 228.8-229.7°C

(c) *Spectroscopy data:* Broad peak at 267.3 nm (E_1^1 85.7)

(d) *Solubility:* Soluble in water (1g in 290 ml), boiling water (1 in 25), acetone (1 in 12), ethanol (1 in 30) and glycerol (1 in 50); slightly soluble in chloroform and in diethyl ether; soluble in dilute aqueous solutions of ammonia and alkaline hydroxides and carbonates

(e) *pH of aqueous solution:* Acid to litmus (National Research Council, 1972)

(f) *Sweetness:* Dilute aqueous solution is about 500 times sweeter than a solution containing an equal concentration by weight of sucrose.

1.4 Technical products and impurities

Saccharin is available in the US as saccharin insoluble powder FCC (Food Chemicals Codex), which meets or exceeds the following specifications: 98-101% active ingredient on an anhydrous basis, a maximum of 100 mg/kg toluenesulphonamides, 30 mg/kg selenium, 10 mg/kg heavy metals (as lead), and 3 mg/kg arsenic. It passes a colour-precipitate test for benzoic and salicylic acids and a colour test for readily carbonizable substances (National Research Council, 1972, 1974; The Sherwin-Williams Co., 1978a).

Various national and international pharmacopoeias give specifications for the purity of saccharin in pharmaceutical products. For example, saccharin is available in the US as a USP grade containing 98-101% active ingredient on an anhydrous basis (US Pharmacopeial Convention, Inc., 1975).

In France, saccharin is available as non-nutritive sweetening tablets containing: (1) 20 mg saccharin, 8 μg disodium methylarsonate (added to reduce its bitter taste), and 0.2 mg lithium chloride; and (2) 25 mg saccharin, 75 mg sodium bicarbonate and 0.15 mg sodium arsenate. No limits have been set on the content of *ortho*-toluenesulphonamide or other impurities in saccharin.

In the Federal Republic of Germany, saccharin meets the following specifications: 98% active ingredient on an anhydrous basis and a maximum of 10 mg/kg each of *ortho*- and *para*-toluenesulphonamides and 30 mg/kg selenium (Bundesminister der Justiz, 1979).

In the UK, no maximum limit for the content of *ortho*-toluenesulphonamide has been regulated at present; however, all existing regulations for non-nutritive sweeteners are under review.

Impurities have been identified in commercial saccharin made by both the Remsen-Fahlberg process (known to be used in Japan, the Republic of Korea and the UK) and the Maumee process (known to be used in the US) (US International Trade Commission, 1977a). Table 1 is a summary of published data on impurities in saccharin and sodium saccharin.

Sodium saccharin

1.1 Synonyms and trade names

Chem. Abstr. Services Reg. No.: 128-44-9

Chem. Abstr. Name: 1,2-Benzisothiazol-3(2*H*)-one, 1,1-dioxide, sodium salt

Synonyms: 1,2-Benzisothiazolin-3-one,1,1-dioxide, sodium salt; saccharin sodium; saccharin soluble; sodium benzosulphimide; sodium 2-benzosulphimide; sodium *ortho*-benzosulphimide; sodium saccharide; sodium saccharinate; sodium saccharine; soluble saccharin; 2-sulphobenzoic imide, sodium salt

Trade names: Cristallose; Crystallose; Dagutan; Kristallose; ODA; Saccharinnatrium; Saccharoidum Natricum; Saxin; Soluble Gluside; Succaril (also contains sodium cyclamate); Sucra; Sweeta; Sykose; Willosetten

1.2 Structural and molecular formulae and molecular weight

$C_7H_4NNaO_3S$ Mol. wt: 205.2

Table 1. Reported impurities in saccharin and sodium saccharin

Impurity	Approx. concentration reported (mg/kg)	Synthetic method[a]	Reference
ortho-Toluenesulphonamide	up to 6000 (before 1973-74)	RF	National Research Council/National Academy of Sciences (1978)
	≤25 (more recently)	RF	National Research Council/National Academy of Sciences (1978)
	⟨0.1	M	Stavrić et al. (1976)
para-Toluenesulphonamide	≤5	RF	Stavrić et al. (1976)
	⟨0.2	M	National Research Council/National Academy of Sciences (1978)
	I[b]	RF	Riggin et al. (1978)
			Stavrić et al. (1976)
1,2-Benzisothiazol-1,1-dioxide	≤10	RF	National Research Council/National Academy of Sciences (1978)
	—	RF	Stavrić et al. (1976)
			Riggin et al. (1978)
1,2-Benzisothiazoline-1,1-dioxide	1 - 10	RF	National Research Council/National Academy of Sciences (1978)
	—	RF	Riggin et al. (1978)
	—	M	Stavrić et al. (1976)
			Riggin et al. (1978)
3-Aminobenzisothiazol-1,1-dioxide	2 - 19	RF	Riggin et al. (1978)
	1	RF	National Research Council/National Academy of Sciences (1978)
	4 - 17	M	Riggin et al. (1978)

Table 1 (contd)

Impurity	Approx. concentration reported (mg/kg)	Synthetic method[a]	Reference
5-Chlorosaccharin	—	RF	National Research Council/National Academy of Sciences (1978)
	⟨25	M	Riggin et al. (1978)
			Riggin et al. (1978)
6-Chlorosaccharin	—	M, RF	National Research Council/National Academy of Sciences (1978)
			Riggin et al. (1978)
Ammonium saccharin	50 - 500	M	Riggin et al. (1978)
Methyl saccharin	0.16	M	Riggin et al. (1978)
Diphenyl sulphone	1 - 7	RF	Riggin et al. (1978)
ortho,ortho'-Ditolylsulphone			
ortho,meta'-Ditolylsulphone			
ortho,para'-Ditolylsulphone	⟨50 (total)	RF	Stavrić et al. (1976); Riggin et al. (1978)
meta,para'-Ditolylsulphone	⟨5 (total)	RF	National Research Council/National Academy of Sciences (1978)
para,para'-Ditolylsulphone			
ortho-Sulphamoylbenzoic acid	0 - 181	RF	Riggin et al. (1978)
	21 - 41	M	Riggin et al. (1978)
para-Sulphamoylbenzoic acid	10 - 1057	RF	Riggin et al. (1978)
	—	M	Riggin et al. (1978)

Table 1 (contd)

Impurity	Approx. concentration reported (mg/kg)	Synthetic method[a]	Reference
ortho-Chlorobenzoic acid	—	M, RF	National Research Council/National Academy of Sciences (1978)
ortho-Sulphobenzoic acid	—	M, RF	Riggin *et al.* (1978)
ortho-Sulphobenzoic acid, ammonium salt	—	M, RF	National Research Council/National Academy of Sciences (1978)
n-Tetracosane	—	RF	Stavrić *et al.* (1976)
			Riggin *et al.* (1978)
Bis(4-carboxyphenyl)sulphone	10	RF	Riggin *et al.* (1978)
Toluene-2,4-disulphonamide	—	RF	National Research Council/National Academy of Sciences (1978)
Saccharin-*ortho*-toluenesulphonamide	—	RF	National Research Council/National Academy of Sciences (1978)
Saccharin-6-sulphonamide	—	RF	National Research Council/National Academy of Sciences (1978)
N-Methyl-*ortho*-toluenesulphonamide	—	RF	National Research Council/National Academy of Sciences (1978)
Methyl-*ortho*-chlorobenzoate	—	RF	National Research Council/National Academy of Sciences (1978)
4,4'-Dibenzoylsulphone	—	RF	National Research Council/National Academy of Sciences (1978)
2- or 3- Carboxy thiaxanthone-5-dioxide	—	RF	National Research Council/National Academy of Sciences (1978)

Table 1 (contd)

Impurity	Approx. concentration reported (mg/kg)	Synthetic method [a]	Reference
ortho-Sulphobenzamide	—	RF	National Research Council/National Academy of Sciences (1978)
Methyl-*ortho*-sulphamoylbenzoate	—	RF	National Research Council/National Academy of Sciences (1978)
Methyl-*N*-methylsulphamoyl-benzoate	—	RF	National Research Council/National Academy of Sciences (1978)
Saccharin-*ortho*-toluene-sulphoxylimide	—	RF	Riggin *et al.* (1978)
Various phthalate esters	0.04	M	Riggin *et al.* (1978)
Trioctyl phosphate	0.06	M	Riggin *et al.* (1978)
Various fatty acid amides	0.75	M	Riggin *et al.* (1978)
Mineral oil (saturated hydro-carbons)	5.0	M	Riggin *et al.* (1978)
Butylated hydroxytoluene	0.04	M	Riggin *et al.* (1978)
Butylated hydroxyanisole	0.01	M	Riggin *et al.* (1978)
Methyl anthranilate	0.05	M	Riggin *et al.* (1978)
ortho-Chlorobenzamide	0.02	M	Riggin *et al.* (1978)
Trichlorobenzene	0.05	M	Riggin *et al.* (1978)
2,6-Di-*tert*-butyl-*para*-benzo-quinone	0.005	M	Riggin *et al.* (1978)

Table 1 (contd)

Impurity	Approx. concentration reported (mg/kg)	Synthetic method[a]	Reference
Lead			
Selenium			
Silver			
Arsenic	Below Food Chemicals Codex specifications (< 0.5)	M	Riggin et al. (1978)
Bismuth			
Cadmium			
Copper			
Mercury			
Tin			

[a]RF - Remsen-Fahlberg method; M - Maumee method

[b]I - Identified but not quantified

1.3 Chemical and physical properties of the dihydrate

From Wade (1977), unless otherwise specified

(a) Description: White crystalline powder with an intensely sweet taste

(b) Melting-point: Greater than 300°C (decomposes) (Beck, 1969)

(c) Solubility: Soluble in water (1g in 1.5 ml) and ethanol (1 in 50)

(d) pH of aqueous solution: Neutral or alkaline to litmus but not alkaline to phenol-phthalein (Windholz, 1976)

(e) Sweetness: Dilute aqueous solution is about 300 times sweeter than a solution containing an equal concentration by weight of sucrose.

1.4 Technical products and impurities

Sodium saccharin FCC (Food Chemicals Codex) is available in the US in four grades: spray-dried, containing 3.0% moisture; powder, containing 5.0-5.8% moisture; pelletized, containing 10.5-11.5% moisture; and granular, containing 14.0-15.0% moisture. Each of these grades meets or exceeds the following Food Chemicals Codex specifications: 98-101% active ingredient on an anhydrous basis, 3-15% water, 100 mg/kg toluenesulphonamides, 30 mg/kg selenium, 10 mg/kg heavy metals (as lead) and 3 mg/kg arsenic. They pass a colour-precipitate test for benzoates and salicylates, a colour test for readily carbonizable substances and a colour test for alkalinity (National Research Council, 1972, 1974; The Sherwin-Williams Co., 1977a, 1978b). An industrial grade is also marketed; however, no specifications were available to the Working Group (The Sherwin-Williams Co., 1977b).

Various national and international pharmacopoeias give specifications for the purity of sodium saccharin in pharmaceutical products. For example, it is available in the US as a National Formulary (NF) grade containing 98-101% active ingredient on an anhydrous basis. Tablets are available in 15, 30 and 60 mg doses which contain 95-110% of the stated amount of sodium saccharin (National Formulary Board, 1975).

Until 1970, when the use of cyclamates in food was banned in the US, sodium saccharin was also available in: (1) aqueous solutions containing about 0.6% sodium saccharin combined with about 6% sodium cyclamate and (2) tablets containing about 5 mg sodium saccharin combined with about 50 mg sodium cyclamate (National Formulary Board, 1970).

Sodium saccharin available in Europe has the following specifications: purity, 98-101% on a dried basis; loss on drying, 15% max; a minimum of 32% sulphate ash on a dried basis; a maximum of 200 mg/kg sulphate, 200 mg/kg chloride, 30 mg/kg selenium, 10 mg/kg heavy metals, 10 mg/kg *ortho*-toluenesulphonamide and 2 mg/kg arsenic; and no visible contamination by a thin-layer chromatographic test.

In France, sodium saccharin is available as a non-nutritive sweetening tablet containing 13 mg sodium saccharin and 20 μg 5-methoxyresorcinol; and a tablet containing 50 mg sodium cyclamate and 5 mg sodium saccharin.

It is available in the UK as an aqueous solution and in 12.5 mg tablets (Wade, 1977).

In the Federal Republic of Germany, sodium saccharin meets the following specifications: 98% active on an anhydrous basis and a maximum of 10 mg/kg *ortho*-toluenesulphonamide and 30 mg/kg selenium (Bundesminister der Justiz, 1979).

In the UK, no maximum limit for the content of *ortho*-toluenesulphonamide in sodium saccharin has been regulated at present; however, all existing regulations for non-nutritive sweeteners are under review.

Sodium saccharin available in Japan must be 99% pure and contain a maximum of 100 mg/kg *ortho*-toluenesulphonamide; the *ortho*-toluenesulphonamide content at present has been found to be in the range of 15-20 mg/kg.

Calcium saccharin

1.1 Synonyms and trade names

Chem. Abstr. Services Reg. No.: 6485-34-3

Chem. Abstr. Name: 1,2-Benzisothiazol-3(2*H*)-one, 1,1-dioxide, calcium salt

Synonyms: 1,2-Benzisothiazolin-3-one,1,1-dioxide, calcium salt; calcium benzosulphimide; calcium 2-benzosulphimide; calcium-*ortho*-benzosulphimide; calcium saccharina; calcium saccharinate; calcium saccharine; saccharin calcium; 2-sulphobenzoic imide, calcium salt

Trade name: Daramin

1.2 Structural and molecular formulae and molecular weight

$C_{14}H_8N_2CaO_6S_2$ Mol. wt: 404.4

1.3 Chemical and physical properties of the hydrate

From Beck (1969) and Wade (1977)

(a) Description: White crystalline powder with intensely sweet taste

(b) Solubility: Soluble in water (1 g in 1.5 ml) and 92% ethanol (1 in 33)

(c) Sweetness: Dilute aqueous solution is about 300 times sweeter than a solution containing an equal concentration by weight of sucrose.

1.4 Technical products and impurities

In 1975, calcium saccharin that met specifications for the US National Formulary (NF) grade was required to contain 98-101% active ingredient on an anhydrous basis, 3-15% water, a maximum of 3 mg/kg arsenic, 30 mg/kg selenium and 10 mg/kg heavy metals, and to pass a colour-precipitate test for benzoates and salicylates and a colour test for readily carbonizable substances (National Formulary Board, 1975).

Until 1970, when the use of cyclamates in food was banned in the US, calcium saccharin was also available in: (1) aqueous solutions containing about 0.6% calcium saccharin combined with about 6% calcium cyclamates, and (2) tablets containing about 5 mg calcium saccharin combined with about 50 mg calcium cyclamate (National Formulary Board, 1970).

ortho-**Toluenesulphonamide**

1.1 Synonyms and trade names

Chem. Abstr. Services Reg. No.: 88-19-7

Chem. Abstr. Name: 2-Methylbenzenesulfonamide

1.2 Structural and molecular formulae and molecular weight

$C_7H_9NO_2S$ Mol. wt: 171.2

1.3 Chemical and physical properties of the pure substance

From Hawley (1977) and Weast (1977), unless otherwise specified

(a) Description: Colourless crystals

(b) Melting-point: 156.3°C

(c) Spectroscopy data: Ultra-violet spectrum has two sharp peaks at 268 and 275 nm (in methanol) (Grasselli, 1973)

(d) Solubility: Soluble in ethanol; slightly soluble in water and diethyl ether

1.4 Technical products and impurities

ortho-Toluenesulphonamide is not produced commercially as a separate chemical in the US; however, a product consisting of a mixture of unknown proportions of the *ortho*- and *para*-isomers of toluenesulphonamide is produced in the US as fine, white-to-light cream granular particles containing 1.0% maximum moisture, with the following properties: flash-point, 215°C; melting-point, 105°C; boiling-point (10 mm), 214°C; and pH, 4.0 min (Monsanto Industrial Chemicals Co., undated).

ortho-Toluenesulphonamide available in Japan has the following specifications: melting-point, 155°C min; water, 0.5% max; ash, 0.2% max; *para*-toluenesulphonamide, 2% max.

2. Production, Use, Occurrence and Analysis

2.1 Production and use

SACCHARIN, SODIUM SACCHARIN AND CALCIUM SACCHARIN

(a) Production

Saccharin was first synthesized in 1879 by Remsen & Fahlberg by: (1) reaction of toluene with chlorosulphonic acid to produce *ortho-* and *para*-toluenesulphonyl chlorides; (2) separation of the *ortho*-isomer followed by treatment with ammonia to form *ortho*-toluenesulphonamide; (3) oxidation to *ortho*-sulphamoylbenzoic acid, which, on heating, was cyclized to saccharin (Remsen & Fahlberg, 1879). Essentially the same method was reportedly used for commercial production by one US company until 1972 and is still used by the six producing companies in Japan, the three producing companies in the Republic of Korea (US International Trade Commission, 1977a) and the sole producer in the UK.

Currently, saccharin and sodium saccharin are produced commercially in the US only by the Maumee process. In this process, methyl anthranilate (made either by the methylation of anthranilic acid, the reaction of phthalic anhydride with ammonia, sodium hypochlorite and methanol, or the reaction of isatoic anhydride with methanol) is diazotized by treatment with sodium nitrite and hydrochloric acid to form 2-carbomethoxybenzenediazonium chloride. Sulphonation of this produces 2-carbomethyoxybenzenesulphinic acid, which is converted to 2-carbomethoxybenzenesulphonyl chloride with chlorine. Amidation of this sulphonylchloride, followed by acidification, forms saccharin, which is treated with either sodium hydroxide or sodium bicarbonate to produce sodium saccharin (National Research Council/National Academy of Sciences, 1978). Calcium saccharin can be produced by the reaction of calcium hydroxide with saccharin.

Saccharin and saccharin sodium have been produced commercially in the US for over 80 years (Crammer & Ikan, 1977); calcium saccharin was first produced commercially in the US in 1953 (US Tariff Commission, 1954). From an estimated level of 180 thousand kg in 1957, US production of saccharin (all forms) increased gradually to an estimated 2040 thousand kg in 1970. Only one US company reported commercial production of an undisclosed amount (see preamble, p. 20) of saccharin and sodium saccharin in 1977 (US International Trade Commission, 1978a); one source has estimated that a total of 2177 thousand kg were produced in that year (National Research Council/National Academy of Sciences, 1978). Commercial production of calcium saccharin was last reported by one company in the US in 1974 (US International Trade Commission, 1976a).

US imports of saccharin (all forms) increased from 45 thousand kg in 1955 to 500 thousand kg in 1963; after decreasing to a low of 310 thousand kg in 1967, imports increased to a high of 1540 thousand kg in 1974. By 1977, US imports of saccharin (all forms), chiefly from Japan (68%) and the Republic of Korea (19%), amounted to 1380 thousand kg (US Department of Commerce, 1978). A total of 214 thousand kg saccharin, 716 thousand kg sodium saccharin and 61 thousand kg calcium saccharin were imported through principal US customs districts in 1977 (US International Trade Commission, 1978b).

Saccharin and sodium saccharin are not produced commercially in Canada; however, they are imported (primarily from the US and Japan).

Annual production of saccharin and sodium saccharin in Europe is estimated to be in the range of 100-1000 thousand kg for each chemical; the Federal Republic of Germany, Spain and the UK are believed to be the major producing countries. Annual saccharin production in the Federal Republic of Germany was 30 thousand kg in 1894, increased to 300 thousand kg in 1922, decreased to 96 thousand kg in 1934, rose to 500 thousand kg in 1944 and dropped again to 27 thousand kg in 1965 (Crampton, 1975). In the UK, commercial production of saccharin and sodium saccharin was first reported in 1916.

Saccharin and sodium saccharin have been produced commercially in Japan since before 1945. In 1978, six Japanese manufacturers produced an estimated 2840 thousand kg each of saccharin and sodium saccharin, and about 1930 thousand kg of sodium saccharin were exported.

Saccharin and sodium saccharin are also produced commercially in Taiwan; however, no information was available on the quantities produced. In 1976, saccharin was produced commercially by three companies in the Republic of Korea (US International Trade Commission, 1977a).

(b)   Use

Saccharin was initially used as a non-nutritive sweetening agent in 1907, but prior to that it had been used as an antiseptic and preservative to retard fermentation in food (National Research Council/National Academy of Sciences, 1978). Since 1970, when the use of cyclamates in food was banned in the US, the food grades of the various forms of saccharin have been used as non-nutritive sweetening agents in a variety of applications (National Formulary Board, 1970, 1975; National Research Council/National Academy of Sciences, 1978).

The US consumption pattern for saccharin (all forms) in 1976 has been estimated as follows: 77% in food uses: 45% in soft drinks, 18% in 'tabletop' sweeteners, and 14% in other foods such as fruits, premixes, juices, sweets, chewing gum and jellies; and 23% in nonfood items: 10% in cosmetics such as toothpaste, mouthwash and lipstick, 7% in pharmaceuticals such as coatings on pills, 2% in smokeless tobacco products such as chewing tobacco and snuff, 2% in electroplating, 1% in cattle feed and 1% in miscellaneous uses (National Research Council/National Academy of Sciences, 1978).

Typical concentrations of sodium saccharin in food products are as follows: sugar substitutes, 13.5 mg/teaspoon sugar sweetening equivalent; carbonated soft drinks, 9.5 mg/ fluid ounce; still soft drinks, 5.5 mg/fluid ounce; jams and jellies, 4.5 mg/teaspoon; chewing gum, 2.2 mg/stick.

It has been reported that saccharin itself (as opposed to its salts) has been used in the sweetening of pharmaceutical tablets and in the processing of tobacco (Anon., 1963).

Industrial grade sodium saccharin is reportedly used as a brightener in nickel-plating baths, as an antistatic agent in plastics and textiles, as a polymer modifier and accelerator in photosensitive dispersions, and as a light fastness aid in nylon dyes (The Sherwin-Williams Co., 1977b)

It has been reported that before 1977 approximately 205 thousand kg of saccharin were consumed in Canada annually for food and industrial uses (Canadian Health & Welfare Department, 1977).

Consumption of saccharin and sodium saccharin in western Europe is estimated to be in the range of 100-1000 and 1000-5000 thousand kg, respectively.

In Japan, saccharin is also used as a chemical intermediate for the fungicide probenazole, which is used commercially in controlling rice blast (Yamada, 1975). Of the estimated 914 thousand kg of saccharin sodium used in Japan in 1978, approximately 60% was used in foods and beverages and 40% in miscellaneous uses (e.g., industrial applications and pharmaceutical uses).

In the US, saccharin (including the calcium, sodium and ammonium salts) was approved for use in foods under the 1958 Food Additives Amendment to the Food, Drug, and Cosmetic Act. Under the provisions of this amendment, saccharin was included in those substances that had been in use prior to 1958 and that had been accorded GRAS (generally recognized as safe) status (National Research Council/National Academy of Sciences, 1978). On 1 February, 1972, questions concerning the safety of saccharin prompted the US Food and Drug Administration (FDA) to remove saccharin from GRAS status and to establish the following interim food additive regulation. The use of saccharin and its sodium, calcium and ammonium salts as sweetening agents in food in the US is permitted, provided the amounts do not exceed the following: 12 mg per oz in beverages and in bases or mixes when prepared for consumption in accordance with directions; 20 mg of additive (calculated as saccharin) for each expressed teaspoonful of sugar sweetening equivalency, as a sugar substitute for cooking or table use; and 30 mg per serving in processed foods. The additives are intended for use in vitamin tablets, chewing gum and in nonstandardized bakery products and must provide labelling, including the name of the additive, concentration (expressed as saccharin) and adequate directions for use (US Food & Drug Administration, 1977a, 1978).

On 7 January 1977, an amendment to the interim food additive regulation for saccharin and its salts was proposed to establish a tolerance for 25 mg *ortho*-toluenesulphonamide per kg saccharin (US Food & Drug Administration, 1977b).

In compliance with the Delaney clause of the amendment, which prohibits the use in food of any ingredient shown to cause cancer in animals or man, the FDA published a proposal to ban the food use of saccharin on 15 April 1977 (US Food & Drug Administration, 1977c). Final regulations by the FDA are now pending additional study as a result of the Saccharin Study and Labeling Act, passed by the US Congress in November 1977. The act requires studies of the impurities and toxicity of saccharin, and of the health benefits, if any, resulting from the use of non-nutritive sweeteners. It also requires certain labels and notices for foods containing saccharin (effective 21 February 1978) and prohibits action restricting the continued use of saccharin as a component of food, drugs and cosmetics for 18 months (Anon., 1978; US Food & Drug Administration, 1978; US International Trade Commission, 1977a).

In 1977, the Joint FAO/WHO Expert Committee on Food Additives re-evaluated the previously established unconditional acceptable daily intake (ADI) of 0-5 mg/kg bw and the conditional ADI of 0-15 mg/kg bw for saccharin and established a temporary acceptable daily saccharin intake of 0-2.5 mg/kg bw until further testing is completed (WHO, 1978).

On 29 March 1978, the Commission of the European Communities recommended to its member states the temporary ADI of 0-2.5 mg/kg bw proposed by the Joint FAO/WHO Expert Committee on Food Additives (Commission of the European Communities, 1978).

The regulatory status of non-nutritive sweeteners containing saccharin and/or cyclamates in various countries is outlined in the Appendix to the **General Remarks on the Substances Considered**, p. 39.

ORTHO-TOLUENESULPHONAMIDE

(a) *Production*

ortho-Toluenesulphonamide was prepared in 1879 by Remsen and Fahlberg by: (1) reaction of toluene with chlorosulphonic acid to produce *ortho*- and *para*-toluenesulphonyl chlorides, and (2) separation of the *ortho*-isomer followed by treatment with ammonia to form *ortho*-toluenesulphonamide (Remsen & Fahlberg, 1879). Essentially the same procedure is believed to have been used for its commercial production in the US and is still used for its commercial production in Japan.

In the US, *ortho*-toluenesulphonamide was produced in commercial quantities from 1921 (US Tariff Commission, 1922) until 1975 (US International Trade Commission, 1977b); and an *ortho,para*-toluenesulphonamide mixture has been produced commercially since 1939 (US Tariff Commission, 1940). Only one US company reported commercial production of an undisclosed amount (see preamble, p. 20) of *ortho*-toluenesulphonamide in 1975 (US International Trade Commission, 1977b) and of *ortho*-, *para*-toluenesulphonamide mixtures in 1977 (US International Trade Commission, 1978a).

In 1973, US imports of *ortho,para*-toluenesulphonamides through the principal US customs districts were reported as 70.2 thousand kg '*ortho,para*-toluenesulphonamide' and 77.1 thousand kg '*ortho,para*-toluenesulphonamide mixtures (Topcizer no.2)' (US Tariff Commission, 1974). In 1974, imports of the latter were reported to have been 18.6 thousand kg (US International Trade Commission, 1976b). No imports have been reported in recent years.

ortho-Toluenesulphonamide is believed to be produced commercially in Italy and The Netherlands; however, no information was available on the quantities produced.

ortho-Toluenesulphonamide has been prepared commercially in Japan since before 1945. In 1978, three Japanese manufacturers produced an estimated 3 million kg *ortho*-toluenesulphonamide and about 2 million kg of the *ortho,para*-toluenesulphonamide mixture.

(b) *Use*

Until 1972, *ortho*-toluenesulphonamide was used in the US as a chemical intermediate for the commercial production of saccharin (US International Trade Commission, 1977a). The *ortho*- and *para*-toluenesulphonamide mixture is used as a reactive plasticizer in hot-melt adhesives to improve the flow properties of thermosetting resins (e.g., melamine, urea and phenolic resins) and to impart flexibility to coatings based on resins made from casein, shellac, zein and soya protein (Monsanto Industrial Chemicals Co., undated). This mixture is also believed to be used as a carrier in fluorescent pigments.

ortho-Toluenesulphonamide is used as a starting material for the commercial production of saccharin in Japan, the Republic of Korea (US International Trade Commission, 1977a) and the UK. In Japan, 60% of the *ortho*-toluenesulphonamide consumed is used as a chemical intermediate for the commercial production of saccharin, and 40% (in the form of the *ortho*- and *para*-toluenesulphonamide mixture) is used as a plasticizer and pigment carrier.

The US Food and Drug Administration has classified the mixture of *ortho*- and *para*-toluenesulphonamides as a safe component of adhesives used in articles intended for packaging, transporting or holding food if used in quantities not exceeding the limits of good manufacturing practice (US Food & Drug Administration, 1978).

(c)   Occurrence

Saccharin, sodium and calcium saccharin and *ortho*-toluenesulphonamide do not occur as natural products.

2.3 Analysis

Typical methods for the analysis of saccharin, sodium saccharin and calcium saccharin are summarized in Table 2; methods for *ortho*-toluenesulphonamide are listed in Table 3.

Table 2. Methods for the analysis of saccharin, sodium saccharin and calcium saccharin

Sample matrix	Sample preparation	Assay procedure	Limit of detection	Reference
Bulk chemical	Dissolve saccharin (hot water), add phenolphthalein	Titration (sodium hydroxide)	-	WHO, 1976
Bulk chemical	Dry saccharin salts, dissolve (acetic acid), add crystal violet-glacial acetic acid	Titration (perchloric acid)	-	WHO, 1976
Pharmaceutical preparations	Add hydrochloric acid, perform series of extractions (isopropyl ether), filter through anhydrous sodium sulphate, evaporate, dissolve (methanol), evaporate, add N,O-bis-(trimethylsilyl)acetamide, add internal standard (n-octacosane)	GC/FID	-	Ratchik & Viswanathan, 1975
Multivitamin tablet	Powder, extract (diethyl ether), add hydrochloric acid, extract (diethyl ether), filter through anhydrous sodium sulphate, evaporate, dissolve (ethanol)	PGC/FID/TCD	3.0 μg	Szinai & Roy, 1976
Liquid sweetener concentrates	Inject directly	HPLC/UV (254 nm)	0.014 μg	Smyly et al., 1976
Sweetener tablets	Powder, dissolve (sodium carbonate solution)	UV (325-220 nm)	-	Hussein et al., 1976
Toothpaste	Dilute (water), centrifuge	HPLC/UV (254 nm)	-	Simko, 1977
Soft drinks	Expel gases, acidify (sulphuric acid), perform series of extractions (diethyl ether) and washings (water), evaporate, add ethanol, copper (II) acetate solution and phenothiazine solution, heat, add ethanol and xylene, dilute (water), agitate, dry xylene layer with anhydrous sodium sulphate	VIS (510 nm)	-	Tanaka et al., 1977

Table 2 (contd)

Sample matrix	Sample preparation	Assay procedure	Limit of detection	Reference
Soft drinks	Expel gases	HPLC/UV (254 nm)	0.014 μg	Smyly et al., 1976
Soft drinks	Extract (ethyl acetate), basify (sodium hydroxide)	MECA (384 nm)	2 mg/l	Belcher et al., 1976
Soft drinks	Expel gases	PGC/FID/TCD	1.0 μg	Szinai & Roy, 1976
Beverages	Acidify (hydrochloric acid), perform series of extractions (chloroform) and washings (water), evaporate, dissolve (sodium carbonate solution)	UV (350-220 nm)	-	Hussein et al., 1976
Sweetened wine	Evaporate, add sulphuric acid, extract (diethyl ether), evaporate, add internal standard (benzenesulphonic acid)	HPLC/UV (254 nm)	25 mg/l	Tenenbaum & Martin, 1977
Chewing gum	Add internal standard (dilute aminobenzoic acid) and toluene, agitate until disintegration, separate aqueous phase, filter	HPLC/UV (254 nm)	-	Eng et al., 1977
Chewing gum	Freeze, pulverize, dilute (water), acidify (hydrochloric acid), perform series of extractions (chloroform) and washings (water), evaporate, dissolve (sodium carbonate solution)	UV (325-220 nm)	-	Hussein et al., 1976
Urine	Add tetrabutylammonium hydrogen sulphate (buffer, pH 7.4), agitate with methyl iodide and dichloromethane, dilute with ethyl acetate, evaporate, add ethyl acetate and saturated silver sulphate solution, agitate	GC/ECD	10 μg/l	Hartvig et al., 1978

Abbreviations: GC/FID - gas chromatography/flame-ionization detection; HPLC/UV - high-pressure liquid chromatography/ultra-violet spectrometry; VIS - visible spectrometry; MECA - molecular emission cavity analysis spectrometry; GC/EC - gas chromatography/electron capture detection; PGC/FID/TCD - pyrolysis gas chromatography/flame-ionization detection/thermal conductivity detection; UV - ultra-violet spectrometry

Table 3. Methods for the analysis of *ortho*-toluenesulphonamide

Sample matrix	Sample preparation	Assay procedure	Limit of detection	Reference
Saccharin or sodium saccharin	Neutralize if acid form (sodium hydroxide), dissolve (water), extract (dichloromethane), add 5% sodium bicarbonate solution, agitate, separate organic phase, evaporate, add methylene chloride	GC/FID	0.05 mg/kg	Janiak *et al.*, 1978
	Neutralize if acid form (15% sodium hydroxide), perform series of extractions (ethyl acetate), evaporate, add internal standard (caffeine, ethyl acetate solution)	GC/FID	0.05 mg/kg	Stavrić *et al.*, 1974
	Neutralize if acid form (sodium hydroxide), add 0.5% disodium hydrogen phosphate, perform series of extractions (dichloromethane), evaporate, add ethanol, concentrate, react residue with TRI-SIL reagent	UV	0.01 mg/ml	Jacin, 1975
Nickel-plating electrolyte	Extract (chloroform), evaporate, dissolve (water), separate by TLC (benzene:ethyl acetate:ethanol, 50:20:1, and diethyl ether:ethyl acetate, 1:1)	EP/TLC (269 nm)	—	Mockute & Bernotiene, 1976

Abbreviations: GC/FID - gas chromatography/flame-ionization detection; UV - ultra-violet spectrometry; EP/TLC - extraction photometry/thin-layer chromatography

3. Biological Data Relevant to the Evaluation
of Carcinogenic Risk to Humans

3.1 Carcinogenicity studies in animals[1]

SACCHARIN AND SODIUM SACCHARIN

(a) Oral administration

Single-generation exposure

Mouse: Groups of 50 female Swiss mice received 0 or 5% saccharin made by the Remsen-Fahlberg method (British Saccharin Sales Co. Ltd, UK) in the diet for 18 months, at which time the survivors were killed. Average survival rates were not affected, and tumour incidences were similar in tested and control animals. No pathological alterations were observed macroscopically in the urinary bladder (Roe *et al.*, 1970) [The Working Group noted that the urinary bladders were not examined histologically].

As part of a multigeneration study, two groups, each of 50 male and 50 female Swiss SPF mice were fed 0.5 or 0.2% saccharin made by the Remsen-Fahlberg method (Bayer Farma NV, The Netherlands; containing 0.5% *ortho*-toluenesulphonamide) for up to 21 months. A concurrent control group of 50 males and 50 females received a standard diet. At 18 months, 62, 64 and 66 animals were still alive in the groups receiving 0.5 and 0.2% saccharin and in the control group, respectively. One control female developed an anaplastic carcinoma of the bladder, and one male in the 0.2% saccharin group had a noninvasive transitional-cell carcinoma of the bladder (Kroes *et al.*, 1977) (see also 'multigeneration exposure', p. 137).

---

[1] The Working Group was aware of completed but unpublished studies on the intragastric administration and feeding of saccharin in the diet to mice; studies in progress on the administration in the diet and drinking-water of sodium saccharin to mice; planned studies on the feeding of sodium saccharin to rats; and completed but as yet unpublished studies on the feeding of sodium saccharin to rats (IARC, 1979).

Groups of 50 male and 50 female dde mice were fed saccharin made by the Remsen-Fahlberg method (purity unspecified) at levels of 0, 0.2, 1.0 or 5% for 21 months. No significant difference in tumour incidence was observed between the treated and untreated groups (National Institute of Hygienic Sciences, 1973).

Groups of 25 male and female Charles River CD mice received sodium saccharin (Merck Co. Ltd, USA & Monsanto Industrial Chemicals Co., USA) in the diet at levels of 0, 1 or 5% for up to 2 years. The Monsanto product contained 345 mg/kg ortho-toluenesulphonamide. Animals that died before 6 months were not examined, and survival times were not reported. Animals were sacrificed when obvious tumours were seen or when they were moribund; all survivors were killed at 2 years. All animals that survived 6 months or longer were examined grossly, and any tissues with abnormal changes were examined histologically; in addition, all vital organs from at least 12 animals in each group were examined histologically. Vascular tumours were seen with increased frequency in the experimental groups, while lung tumours, hepatomas and lymphomas occurred with apparently equal incidence in control and experimental groups. Any differences in incidence of tumours were not considered to be significant and were reported to be absent in a duplicate experiment; however, no data on the duplicate study were given (Homburger, 1978) [The Working Group noted the inadequate reporting of the experiment].

Rat: Groups of 10 male and 10 female Osborne-Mendel rats received 0, 1 and 5% saccharin (source and purity unspecified) in the diet for up to 2 years. Mortality in pooled controls was 14% at 1 year and 68% at 2 years; surviving animals at 1 year were 7 males and 9 females in the 0 dose group, 10 males and 10 females in the 1% group and 9 males and 9 females in the 5% group; no data were given for 2-year survival rates. Seven/18 animals (sex not specified) in the 5% group developed abdominal lymphosarcomas; 4 of the 7 also had thoracic lymphosarcomas. Urinary bladders were not examined (Fitzhugh et al., 1951) [The Working Group noted the small number of animals in each group].

Groups of 20 male and 20 female Boots-Wistar rats were fed 0, 0.005%, 0.05% or 5% saccharin made by the Remsen-Fahlberg method (Boots & Co., UK; purity unspecified) for 2 years. At 18 months, 15 male and 14 female controls, and 10 male and 10 female rats at the highest dose level were still alive. No statistically significant differences in tumour incidence were found between treated and control animals. Only five bladders, all from animals in the highest dose group, were examined histologically. Urothelial hyperplasia was found in 1 male and 1 female, and a bladder papilloma was found in another female. Bladder parasites were not found (Lessel, 1971).

Groups of 52 male and 52 female BD rats were fed 0, 0.2 or 0.5% sodium saccharin made by the Remsen-Fahlberg method (Bayer-Werken AG, FRG; purity unspecified) for up to 30 months, starting between 70 and 90 days of age (average total doses, 0, 83 and 210 g/kg bw). Survival at 18 months was 55/104 controls, 50/104 animals treated with 0.2%

saccharin and 41/104 animals treated with 0.5% saccharin; at 24 months survival was 6/104, 3/104 and 5/104, respectively. Sixteen percent of all animals had parasites (*Strongyloides capillaria*) in the urinary tract. Benign and malignant mesenchymal tumours were found with a similar frequency in all groups. No bladder tumours were observed (Schmähl, 1973).

Groups of 60 male and 60 female Charles River CD rats were fed diets containing sodium saccharin made by the Remsen-Fahlberg method (Daiwa Chemical Co. Ltd, Japan; purity conformed to USP, BP & FCC specifications) for 26 months, to give daily intakes of 0, 0.09, 0.27, 0.81 or 2.43 g/kg bw. Saccharin treatment did not affect survival of female rats: at 18 months, approximately 50% of the original animals were alive. In male rats, survival was affected in a dose-related manner: thus, at 18 months about 80% of male control rats were alive, but only about 50% of those in the highest dose group survived. By 24 months about 10% of the animals were alive in all groups. A total of 4 transitional-cell tumours of the bladder were found, one in a male and one in a female given 0.09 g/kg bw and two in males fed 0.81 g/kg bw; an angiosarcoma of the bladder was found in a male control. Bladder calculi were recorded, but there was no association between the presence of calculi, saccharin treatment and/or bladder tumours. The animals were free from bladder parasites. The combined incidences of lymphomas and leukaemias was 7/54 in males at the highest dose of saccharin and 2/57 in untreated male controls (Munro *et al.*, 1975).

It was reported in an abstract that groups of 54-56 male Wistar rats were fed 0 or 2.5 g/kg bw per day sodium saccharin (source and purity unspecified) for up to 28 months. Ten to 16 rats of each group were killed at 12 months, 11 of each group at 24 months and all survivors (number unspecified) at 28 months. No urinary bladder tumours were observed (Furuya *et al.*, 1975) [The Working Group noted the incomplete reporting of this experiment].

Groups of Charles River CD male and female rats of unspecified size received saccharin (source and purity unspecified) by an unspecified route (in the diet; or by gastric intubation thrice weekly) for 18 months, followed by a 6-month period of observation. A high incidence of benign tumours of the pituitary and mammary glands was found in surviving controls and experimental animals. Survival times, types of pathological examination, tumour types and other important experimental details were omitted (Ulland *et al.*, 1973) [The Working Group noted the inadequacy of this experiment].

Groups of 25 male Charles River CD-1 rats received sodium saccharin (Merck Co. Ltd, USA & Monsanto Industrial Chemicals Co., USA) in the diet at levels of 0, 1 or 5% for up to 2 years. The Monsanto product contained 345 mg/kg *ortho*-toluenesulphonamide. Animals that died before 6 months were not examined, and survival times were not reported. Animals were sacrificed when obvious tumours were seen or when they were moribund; all survivors were killed at 2 years. All animals that survived 6 months or longer were examined grossly, and any tissues with abnormal changes were examined histologically; in addition, all vital organs from at least 12 animals in each group were examined histologically. Tumours of the urinary bladder, pituitary, breast and subcutaneous tissue were seen with equal incidence in all groups (Homburger, 1978) [The Working Group noted the inadequate reporting of the experiment]. Ova consistent with the presence of *Trichosomoides crassicauda* were found in approximately one third of all urines examined from animals in the above experiment. Their presence was not correlated with the occurrence of bladder lesions (Bio-Research Consultants, Inc., 1973).

A group of 75 male and 50 female Wistar SPF rats received sodium saccharin made by the Remsen-Fahlberg method and containing 698 mg/kg *ortho*-toluenesulphonamide (Boots & Co., UK) in the drinking-water to give a daily intake of 2 g/kg bw saccharin. Another group of 75 male and 75 females received 4 g/kg bw per day saccharin in the diet. Controls were 55 males and 50 females. The males receiving saccharin in the drinking-water were also given 1% ammonium chloride for 4 weeks then 0.5% for life, in order to correct a treatment-associated rise in urinary pH. Of the male controls, 25 were given ammonium chloride at the same concentrations. No treatment-associated change in urinary pH occurred in either of the treated groups of females or in males receiving saccharin in the diet. The experiment was terminated after 2 years. Survival at 18 months was 49/55 male and 43/50 female untreated controls, 65/75 males and 44/50 females that received saccharin in the drinking-water, and 55/75 males and 52/75 females fed saccharin in the diet. At 2 years, 37/55 male and 13/50 female controls, 49/75 males and 29/50 females receiving saccharin in the drinking-water, and 12/75 males and 16/75 females fed saccharin in the diet were still alive. In control animals, the total tumour incidence was 1/52 in males and 9/46 in females. In rats receiving saccharin in the drinking-water (2 g/kg bw/day), incidence was 11/71 in males and 10/44 in females; while in rats fed saccharin (4 g/kg bw/day), it was 10/70 in males and 7/68 in females. Transitional-cell carcinomas of the urothelium were not seen in male or female controls, but accounted for 1/71 in males (in the ureter) and 1/44 in females (in the renal pelvis) in rats receiving saccharin in the drinking-water, and 3/70 in males (all in the bladder) and 0/68 in females in the saccharin-fed group. The incidence of lymphosarcomas and/or leukaemia was 0/52 in males and 0/46 in female controls, 4/71 in males and 1/44 in females given saccharin in the drinking-water, and 2/70 in male and 1/68 in female saccharin-fed rats. One Leydig-cell tumour was found in each of the saccharin-treated groups of males, but none occurred in the testes of untreated male controls. There was a treatment-associated increase in microcalculi within the renal tubules of male (but not female) saccharin-treated rats, with an incidence of 2/52 in controls, 30/71 in males given saccharin in the drinking-water and 16/70 in saccharin-fed males. The animals were free from bladder parasites (Chowaniec & Hicks, 1979).

Groups of 50 male and 50 female 30-day old Charles-River CD rats were fed either a control diet or a diet containing 5% sodium saccharin prepared by the Maumee process (The Sherwin-Williams Co., USA) and free of *ortho*-toluenesulphonamide. Survival was not affected by treatment. Bladder tumours (benign and malignant) were observed in 1/36 control males and in 7/38 male rats fed saccharin which survived 87 weeks or more (the time at which the first tumour was observed (P=>0.05). In addition, 1 treated male and 2 treated females had urothelial tumours of the kidney pelvis and 1 treated male had a urethral tumour; no other urothelial tumours were observed in controls. The incidence of bladder calculi was not related to treatment or to tumour incidence. The animals were free of bladder parasites (Arnold et al., 1977, 1980) [The experiment was part of a two-generation study, see p. 138].

A group of 50 female Wistar rats were given 2.0 g/kg bw per day sodium saccharin made by the Maumee process (The Sherwin-Williams Co., USA) in the diet for 2 years. A group of 63 animals served as controls. At week 84, 50/63 controls and 37/50 saccharin-fed rats were still alive. Overall tumour incidences were similar in the two groups; no bladder neoplasms occurred in either group. Mild focal urothelial hyperplasia was seen in one rat fed saccharin. The animals were free from bladder parasites (Hooson et al., 1980) [The Working Group noted that the animals were not started on the test at weaning but had been fed a normal diet for several weeks prior to the start of the study].

Hamster: Groups of 30 male and 30 female random-bred Syrian golden hamsters received saccharin made by the Maumee process (Sigma Chemical Co., USA) at levels of 0, 0.156, 0.312, 0.625 and 1.25% in drinking-water for their natural lifespan. The highest dose level used in this study was the maximum tolerated dose as determined in an 8-week study. The average daily consumption ranged from 44 mg/animal given the 0.156% level to 353 mg/animal given the 1.25% level. The mean survival time was 50-60 weeks in all groups. Pathological changes as well as distribution and histological types of neoplasms were within the range of tumours that occur commonly in hamsters in this colony (Althoff et al., 1975).

Monkey: In an abstract, it was reported that sodium saccharin made by the Remsen-Fahlberg method (Squibb Co., USA, containing 2.4 mg/kg *ortho*-toluenesulphonamide; and Pfaltz & Bauer, Inc., USA, containing 3.2 mg/kg *ortho*-toluenesulphonamide) (Coulston et al., 1975) was given orally at doses of 20, 100 or 500 mg/kg bw per day on 6 days a week to groups of 2, 2 and 3 *Macaca mulatta* (rhesus) monkeys of each sex, respectively. Three animals of each sex served as controls. After 79 months on this regime, 6 male and 6 female monkeys remained in the treated groups; at this time all remaining monkeys were autopsied. Histopathological examination revealed no abnormal pathology in the urinary bladder, kidneys or testis in those surviving the treatment or in those that died during the test (McChesney et al., 1977).

In a study in progress, now in its ninth year, 10 monkeys of 4 different strains are fed 25 mg/kg bw per day sodium saccharin (Fisher Scientific, USA; 'purified'; method of manufacture unspecified) on 5 days per week. Clinical observation has failed to demonstrate any evidence of gross neoplasia; none of the animals have died (Sieber & Adamson, 1978) [The Working Group noted the fact that this study is not yet completed].

Multigeneration exposure

In these studies, animals of each sex of the parent (Fo) generation were fed saccharin from weaning (or very soon after weaning) throughout both pregnancy and the preweaning of their offspring. The offspring were placed on the same diet as their parents for their entire lifespan; thus, their exposure to saccharin was increased by comparison with that of the Fo generation, by the length of the gestation and suckling periods.

Mouse: Saccharin containing 0.5% *ortho*-toluenesulphonamide (Bayer Farma NV, The Netherlands) was fed to groups of Swiss SPF mice in a multigeneration study for life at levels of 0, 0.2 and 0.5% in the diet. The F_0, F3b and F6a generations, consisting of 50 males and 50 females, were used to test the compound for carcinogenicity. The experiments were terminated at 21 months. The survival rates at 18 months were: 66, 62, 64 (F_0: control, 0.5%, 0.2%); 61, 54, 53 (F3b: control, 0.5%, 0.2%); and 67, 48, 54 (F6a: control, 0.5%, 0.2%). Histopathological examination showed that pathological alterations were equally distributed throughout the control and experimental groups. Two male mice, one of the F_0 generation receiving 0.2% saccharin and one of the F3b generation receiving 0.5% saccharin, developed transitional-cell carcinomas of the bladder at 20.5 months. One female control mouse of the F_0 generation had an anaplastic carcinoma of the bladder at 20.5 months (Kroes *et al.*, 1977).

Rat: Groups of 20 male and 20 female weanling Sprague-Dawley rats of the F_1 generation were fed sodium saccharin made by the Remsen-Fahlberg method (source unspecified) at levels of 0, 0.05, 0.5 and 5% of the basal diet for up to 100 weeks. Of F_1 males, 12, 10, 11 and 15 in the respective dosage groups survived to 80 weeks, by comparison with 16, 14, 14 and 19 F_1 females. Seven transitional-cell carcinomas of the urinary bladder developed, all in F_1 males on the 5% saccharin diet (P=0.001). The presence or absence of bladder parasites was not recorded. The total numbers of tumour-bearing animals were: at 0%, 2 males and 8 females; at 0.05%, 1 male and 6 females; at 0.5%, 1 male and 5 females; and at 5.0%, 7 males and 13 females (Tisdel *et al.*, 1974).

Groups of 48 male and 48 female Charles River CD rats of the F_1 generation were fed dietary levels of 0, 0.01, 0.1, 1.0, 5.0 or 7.5% sodium saccharin (method of production and source unspecified) for 28 months. Their parents had been fed the same diet from weaning. There were no significant differences in survival between treated and control animals. Although no difference in bladder cancer incidence was found between F_1 males fed 5% saccharin (1/21) and the F_1 controls (1/25) surviving beyond 18 months, 6/23 F_1 male rats fed 7.5% saccharin developed transitional-cell carcinomas of the bladder. This result was significantly different from that in controls [P=0.018]. There was no apparent correlation between tumour incidence and presence of bladder stones. The bladders were reported to be 'free of visible parasites' (Taylor & Friedman, 1974; US Department of Health, Education, & Welfare, 1973a, b)

Groups of 50 male and 50 female 30-day old Sprague-Dawley rats were fed either a control diet or a diet containing 5% sodium saccharin continuously for life. The saccharin was prepared by the Maumee process (The Sherwin-Williams Co., USA) and was free of *ortho*-toluenesulphonamide. After 3 months on test the animals were mated on a one-to-one basis. All litters were culled to 8 pups (4 males and 4 females) 4 days post-partum in a random manner. The pups were weaned onto their parents' diet, and 50 males and 50 females from each group were randomly selected to constitute the second generation. Survival in the offspring (F_1 generation) was not affected by treatment. Of the F_1 generation animals surviving 67 weeks or longer, at which time the first tumour was observed, none of the 42 male controls but 12 of the 45 saccharin-treated males had developed bladder cancer [P=0.002]. In addition, 1 male had a urethral tumour, and 2 of the 49 surviving females fed 5% sodium saccharin also had bladder cancers. Although urinary bladder calculi were noted occasionally, the incidence of these calculi was not related to the saccharin treatment nor were they associated with the tumours. The animals were free of bladder parasites (see also p.136)(Arnold *et al.*, 1977, 1980).

(b)   Skin application

Mouse: A total dose of 0.24 g saccharin, made by the Remsen-Fahlberg method (British Drug Houses, UK) as an 8% solution in acetone was applied thrice weekly to the skin of 'S' strain mice. Twenty-five days after starting the treatment, the animals were given 18 weekly applications of 0.17% croton oil in acetone. At the end of the croton-oil treatment, a total of 14 skin tumours were observed in 7 of the 20 saccharin-treated animals, by comparison with 4 papillomas in 4 of 19 controls treated with croton oil only. The increase was not statistically significant (Salaman & Roe, 1956).

(c)   Intraperitoneal administration

Mouse: In a test system designed as a short-term whole animal bioassay in which the development of lung tumours was used as an indication of carcinogenicity, groups of 20 female A/He mice were injected intraperitoneally with 0.1 ml of saccharin (Monsanto Industrial Chemicals Co., USA; purity unspecified) in water, three times a week for 8 weeks. Two dose levels were used, to give total doses of 78 g/kg bw (approx. 3.3 g/kg bw per day) and 15.6 g/kg bw (approx. 0.6 g/kg bw per day). The experiment was terminated after 21 weeks. As controls, 30 females were given water intraperitoneally three times a week for 8 weeks and killed after 24 weeks. Saccharin was negative as assessed by the pulmonary tumour response (Stoner *et al.*, 1973) [The Working Group noted the limitations of a negative result obtained from this test system, see General Remarks on the Substances Considered, Vol. 20, p. 34].

(d)   Other experimental systems

Bladder insertion (implantation): Saccharin (source and purity unspecified) (2 mg) was mixed with 4 times its weight of cholesterol. Pellets (9 - 11 mg) containing saccharin were then inserted into the urinary bladder lumina of 20 'stock' *mice* (sex and age unspecified).

An identical group composed of 28 mice received 9-11 mg pellets of cholesterol. The experiment lasted 52 weeks. Of mice that lived 30 weeks, 4/13 saccharin-treated and 1/24 control animals developed bladder cancer (P=0.01) (Allen *et al.*, 1957).

Sodium saccharin (analytically pure; Abbott Laboratories, USA) (4-5 mg) was mixed with 4 times its weight of cholesterol. Pellets (20-24 mg) containing sodium saccharin were then inserted into the urinary bladder lumina in 2 separate trials using groups each composed of 100 female Swiss *mice* aged 60-90 days. Ninety-nine percent of the sodium saccharin disappeared from the pellet within 1.5 days. Identical groups received 20-24 mg pellets of pure cholesterol. The experiment lasted 56 weeks. Only the bladders of animals surviving more than 25 weeks were examined microscopically. The first urinary bladder carcinoma was seen in a saccharin-treated animal 42 weeks after surgical insertion. The overall incidences of bladder carcinomas were 31/66 (trial 1) and 33/64 (trial 2) in saccharin-treated mice as compared with 8/63 (trial 1) and 5/43 (trial 2) in animals exposed to pure cholesterol pellets (P<0.001). The carcinomas in saccharin-exposed mice were more frequently multiple and invasive (P<0.009). They were composed of cells with a high mitotic index and exhibited more squamous or glandular metaplasia than was found in tumours in control animals. No other tissues demonstrated a tumour incidence deviant from the rate seen in control mice (Bryan *et al.*, 1970) (cf. sodium cyclamate, p. 74).

(e)   Administration in conjunction with known carcinogens

Benzo[a]*pyrene (BP):* Groups of 50 female Swiss *mice* received an initial single gastric instillation of 0.2 ml polyethylene glycol either alone or containing 50 μg BP (purities unspecified). Seven days later, the test diet, containing 5% saccharin (British Saccharin Sales Co. Ltd, UK; purity unspecified) was fed for 72 weeks. Average survival rates were not different from those in controls. Although mice treated with BP showed an increased incidence of tumours of the forestomach (20/61), saccharin did not enhance the occurrence (10/32). Hepatocellular adenomas, pulmonary neoplasms and malignant lymphomas occurred with similar frequencies in all groups. No pathological alterations were observed macroscopically in the urinary bladder (Roe *et al.*, 1970) [The Working Group noted that BP is not organotropic for the bladder and that the urinary bladders were not examined histologically].

2-Acetylaminofluorene (AAF): Two groups of 12 Horton Sprague-Dawley female *rats* were fed a diet supplemented with 300 mg AAF/kg of diet for 40 weeks. The test group received in addition 5% sodium saccharin (Abbott Laboratories, USA) in the diet. Eleven of the 12 AAF-fed controls developed palpable mammary and ear-duct tumours in the 40-week period, compared with 6/12 rats fed AAF plus saccharin. In addition, liver tumours were observed in both groups but they were smaller and less malignant in the saccharin-fed animals. Microscopic examination of the urinary bladders indicated that the mucosal lining was hyperplastic in all rats fed AAF and was particularly so in those fed AAF plus saccharin; one animal in the test groups exhibited squamous metaplasia and precancerous changes of the mucosal epithelium. No malignant lesions of the urinary bladder were observed in any of the rats (Ershoff & Bajwa, 1974) [The Working Group noted the inadequate number of animals and the fact that food consumption was not measured, so that it was not possible to assess the intake of AAF or saccharin].

N-*Nitroso*-N-*methylurea (NMU):* A group of 50 female Wistar SPF *rats,* 6-8 weeks of age, were pretreated with 1.5 mg NMU, then 2 days later were administered 4 g/kg bw per day sodium saccharin (Boots Co., UK; Remsen-Fahlberg, containing an average of 698 mg/ kg *ortho*-toluenesulphonamide) in the drinking-water for life or up to 2 years; 50 further females were pretreated with 2 mg NMU and then fed 2 g sodium saccharin/kg bw per day in the diet. NMU (purity unspecified) was dissolved in 0.9% sodium chloride (pH 7.0) and instilled into the bladder. Control groups consisted of 55 male and 50 female untreated rats, 75 males and 50 females given 2 g sodium saccharin /kg bw per day in drinking-water and 75 males and 75 females fed 4 g sodium saccharin/kg bw per day in the diet. For con-current NMU controls, 85 males and females were given 1.5 mg NMU, and 50 were given 2 mg NMU and maintained on a saccharin-free diet for 2 years. The incidences of transitional-cell neoplasms of the bladder in surviving animals whose bladders were examined histologi-cally were: untreated controls, 0/52 males and 0/46 females; lower dose of sodium sacc-harin alone in drinking-water, 0/71 males and 0/44 females; higher dose of sodium sacch-harin alone in diet, 3/70 males and 0/68 females; NMU-treated males and females (1.5 and 2.0 mg) 0/124; NMU followed by the lower dose of sodium saccharin in drinking-water, 23/49 females (47%; $P<0.0005$); NMU followed by the higher dose of sodium saccharin in the diet, 27/47 females (52%; $P<0.0005$). The first bladder tumour was seen after 95 weeks in the saccharin-fed control group and after 8 weeks in the NMU-initiated and sacc-harin-treated test groups. The animals were free from bladder parasites (Chowaniec & Hicks, 1979; Hicks *et al.,* 1978).

A single dose of 2 mg NMU (German Cancer Research Center, FRG) was instilled into the urinary bladder of female Wistar rats (AF-Han strain) (weighing 195 g). Thereafter, 50 animals were given 2% saccharin (The Sherwin-Williams Co., USA; purity unspecified) in the diet, increased after 10 weeks to 4%, for life (1.4-2.5 g/kg bw per day). Control groups consisted of 100 untreated female rats, 50 females receiving NMU alone and 50 females re-ceiving distilled water. A further group of 50 female rats treated with NMU were given 3% calcium carbonate in the diet instead of saccharin. Survival at two years was: controls, 59/100; water controls, 28/50; NMU-treated, 13/50; NMU + calcium carbonate-treated, 15/50; and NMU + saccharin-treated, 14/50. In the NMU-treated groups, the first tumour of the urinary bladder was found after 14 weeks. Urethelial neoplasms (benign and mali-gnant) occurred in the renal pelvis, ureter and urinary bladder. The overall incidences of urinary tract tumours were 57% (NMU only; survival 76 ± 29 weeks), 65% (NMU + sacc-harin; survival, 78 ± 25 weeks) and 65% (NMU + calcium carbonate; survival, 86 ± 23 weeks). In the renal pelvis, frequencies were 28, 57 and 43%; the ureter showed incidences of 17, 12 and 11%; and the urinary bladder had frequencies of 39, 31 and 39%, respectively. Calcifications in the urinary tract, including stone formation, were similar in all treated groups, including water controls; they did not correlate with tumour occurrences. In the untreated controls, as well as in controls receiving a water instillation into the urinary bladder, a tumour of the urinary tract was found. The presence or absence of bladder parasites was not reported   (Mohr *et al.*, 1978) [The Working Group noted that many tumours were found and that the animals were heavier than those used in the experiment by Hicks *et al.*, 1978].

Three groups of 63 female Wistar *rats* were pretreated with 0.15 ml of a saturated solution of NMU (purity unspecified) in saline instilled into the bladder. Two weeks later, rats were given 0 or 2.0 g/kg bw per day sodium saccharin in the drinking-water for 2 years ; one group received saccharin prepared by the Maumee process (The Sherwin-Williams Co., USA) and the second group received saccharin prepared by the Remsen-Fahlberg method (Boots Co., UK) containing 40 mg/kg *ortho*-toluenesulphonamide. At week 84, 22 controls, 43 animals given 'Maumee' sodium saccharin, and 37 rats given 'Remsen-Fahlberg' sodium saccharin had died. An increase in the number of proliferative bladder lesions occurred in animals treated with NMU plus saccharin. The incidence of bladder neoplasia was not significantly different in the saccharin-treated groups, but the latent period was shorter (55 and 52 weeks *versus* 87 weeks).   The animals were free from bladder parasites (Hooson *et al.*, 1980) [The Working Group noted that the animals were not started on the test at weaning but had been fed a normal diet for several weeks prior to the start of the study].

N-[4-(5-Nitro-2-furyl)-2-thiazolyl] formamide (FANFT): Male Fischer *rats*, 4-weeks-old at the start of the experiment, were treated as follows: Group 1, 0.2% FANFT (Sober Laboratories, USA) in powdered diet for 6 weeks, followed immediately by 5% sodium saccharin (Sigma Chemical Co., USA; containing <0.03 mg/kg *ortho*-toluenesulphonamide) in powdered diet for 83 weeks, then standard diet; Group 2, pretreatment with FANFT as Group 1, followed by 6 weeks on standard diet, then 5% sodium saccharin diet for 77 weeks, then standard diet; Group 3, normal diet for 6 weeks, followed by 5% sodium saccharin diet for 83 weeks, then standard diet; Group 4, pretreatment with FANFT as Group 1, followed by standard diet for 98 weeks; and Group 5, untreated controls fed standard diet for 104 weeks. Each group consisted of 20 animals, apart from the control group which had 42 animals. The experiment was terminated after 104 weeks, at which time 6/20, 9/20, 19/20, 16/20 and 27/42 animals survived in groups 1-5, respectively. The incidences of urothelial carcinomas were 18/19 and 13/18 in the FANFT plus saccharin groups, 0/20 in the group receiving saccharin alone, 4/20 in the group receiving FANFT alone, and 0/42 in the untreated controls. In addition, 1/19 animals in Group 1 and 1/18 in Group 2 (FANFT plus saccharin-treated animals) had urinary bladder sarcomas, and 1/20 in Group 4 (FANFT only) had a bladder papilloma. The presence or absence of bladder parasites was not reported (Cohen *et al.*, 1979).

SACCHARIN/CYCLAMATE MIXTURES

(a)   Oral administration

Single-generation exposure

Rat: Two groups of 52 male and 52 female Sprague-Dawley rats, between 70 and 90 days of age, were given a 10:1 mixture of sodium cyclamate:sodium saccharin (Bayer-Werken AG, FRG) daily in the diet for up to 30 months. The cyclamate in the mixture contained less than 4 mg/kg cyclohexylamine;   no information on the purity of the saccharin was given. The mixture was administered at doses of 2 and 5%. An identical group served as controls. At 24 months, approximately 10% of the initial number of animals were still alive. Except for the occurrence of bladder parasites (*Strongyloides capillaria*) in 16% of animals, all examinations were negative. A similar frequency of benign neoplasms occurred in all groups (fibromas, fibroadenomas or adenomas of the mammary gland in females and thymomas in males) (Schmähl, 1973).

It was reported in an abstract that 2 groups of 54-56 Wistar rats received 0 or 2.5 g/kg bw per day of a mixture of sodium cyclamate:sodium saccharin (10:1) (source and purity unspecified) in the diet for 28 months. Ten to 16 rats of each group were killed at 12 months, 11 at 24 months and all survivors at 28 months. No treated or control animals developed tumours of the urinary bladder (Furuya *et al.*, 1975) [The Working Group noted the incomplete reporting of this experiment] .

Groups of 35 male and 45 female FDRL strain Wistar-derived weanling rats were fed a 10:1 mixture of sodium cyclamate:saccharin (Abbott Laboratories, USA; purity and method of manufacture unspecified) in the diet at doses of 0, 500, 1120 and 2500 mg/kg bw per day for 2 years. From week 79 the original dose groups were split, and 50% of the survivors in each group, except the untreated controls, received in addition cyclohexylamine hydrochloride in the diet. The 500 mg group received 25 mg, the 1120 mg group 56 mg, and the 2500 mg group received 125 mg cyclohexylamine/kg bw per day. Mortality rates were similar in control and test groups. Treatment-related pathological changes were seen only in the kidney and bladder. Pelvic hyperplasia was observed more often in the treated groups (8/80, 21/80 and 16/80, as compared with 3/80 in controls). Among animals surviving more than 49 weeks, 9/25 male and 3/35 female rats at the 2500 mg/kg bw dose, compared with 0/35 male and 0/45 female controls, developed transitional-cell carcinomas of the urinary bladder. Of these, 3 male and 2 female rats had received cyclohexylamine. Two of the bladder carcinoma-bearing animals had calculi; 18 rats at this dose level had nonmalignant proliferative bladder lesions. In the lower dose groups, nonmalignant proliferative lesions were found, but their incidence was not significantly higher than that in controls. Renal calcification was seen in 7/12 rats with bladder carcinomas; *Trichosomoides crassicauda* infection was present in one rat with bladder cancer and 4 rats with non-neoplastic proliferative lesions at the highest dose level, in 4 given the 1120 mg/kg dose, in 2 given the 500 mg/kg dose and in 5 control animals (Oser *et al.*, 1975; Price *et al.*, 1970).

Multigeneration exposure

Mouse: In a multigeneration study, a 10:1 mixture of sodium cyclamate:saccharin (5 or 2% and 0.5 or 0.2%, respectively; Bayer Farma NV, The Netherlands) was fed continuously to Swiss SPF mice over 6 generations. The saccharin contained 0.5% *ortho*-toluenesulphonamide; the cyclamate contained 2.1 mg/kg cyclohexylamine. The F_0 (parental) , F3b and F6a generations, consisting of 50 males and 50 females each, were used for the carcinogenicity studies and were treated for 84 weeks. Pathological alterations and urinary bladder calculi occurred with similar frequencies in control and treated groups. Four neoplasms of the urinary bladder occurred: three anaplastic carcinomas (1 in a female control of the F_0 generation and 2 in females of the F_0 and F6a generations fed 0.2% saccharin plus 2% cyclamate) and one papilloma (in a male of the F6a generation given 0.2% saccharin and 2% cyclamate). The mean latent period was more than 80 weeks (Kroes *et al.*, 1977).

ORTHO-TOLUENESULPHONAMIDE

(a)   Oral administration

Rat: In a two-generation study, groups of Charles River CD rats (30 days old) were fed one of the following diets with tap-water *ad libitum:* control; 2.5, 25 or 250 mg/kg bw per day *ortho*-toluenesulphonamide; or 250 mg/kg bw per day *ortho*-toluenesulphonamide with 1% ammonium chloride in the drinking-water. The *ortho*-toluenesulphonamide (Monsanto Industrial Chemicals Co., USA) was more than 99.9% pure.   Each group contained 50 males and 50 females, except for the group receiving ammonium chloride in the drinking-water, which comprised 40 males and 38 females. The F_0 animals were started on test at 32 days of age. After 3 months on test, the animals were mated on a one-to-one basis; all litters were culled to 8 pups (4 males and 4 females) 4 days post partum in a random manner. The pups were weaned onto their parents' diet, and 50 males and 50 females from each group were randomly selected to constitute the second generation (F_1). The two generations remained on test for 30 (F_1) and 32 (F_0) months. The animals were free of bladder parasites. Rats from both generations fed diets providing 250 mg/kg bw or 250 mg/kg bw plus 1% ammonium chloride in the drinking-water had lowered feed consumption. There were no treatment-related effects associated with longevity. The numbers of bladder tumours (all of which were benign) were: in the F_0 generation males - 1 in a control and 1 in each of the 2.5 and 250 mg/kg bw per day *ortho*-toluenesulphonamide groups; females - 1 in the 2.5 mg/kg bw group; in the F_1 generation females - 2 in the 2.5 mg/kg bw group (Arnold *et al.*, 1977, 1980).

Groups of 38 male and 38 female Sprague-Dawley rats, 3 months of age, were administered daily doses of 0, 20 or 200 mg/kg bw *ortho*-toluenesulphonamide (source and purity unspecified) for lifetime by adjusting concentrations added to the diet. Average survivals were 700 days for controls, 770 days for low-dose and 840 days for high-dose animals. The total incidences of malignant tumours were no different in treated groups compared with controls.   Lymphosarcomas developed in 7/71 controls, 10/75 low-dose and 10/76 high-dose animals.   In addition, 3/76 leukoses occurred at the high dose and 5/75 at the low dose, compared with 0/71 in controls.   In high-dose animals, 1/76 carcinoma and 4/76 papillomas of the bladder were found after 759-996 days [P=0.03] ; in low-dose rats, 3/75 papillomas of the bladder occurred after 539, 766 and 873 days.   No bladder tumours occurred in 71 controls (Schmähl, 1978) [The presence or absence of bladder parasites was not recorded and the sexes of animals with bladder tumours were not specified] .

Three groups of 50 or 63 female Wistar rats were administered *ortho*-toluene-sulphonamide (Monsanto Industrial Chemicals Co., USA; pure) at levels of 0 or 0.1% in the drinking-water or 90 mg/kg in the diet for 2 years. Survival was similar in all groups at 84 weeks.   No difference in overall tumour incidence was observed between control and test groups.   No bladder tumours were observed in any group.   Mild diffuse urothelial hyperplasia was found in 1/50 rats fed *ortho*-toluenesulphonamide in the diet (Hooson *et al.*, 1980).

(b)   Administration in conjunction with known carcinogens

N-*Nitroso*-N-*methylurea (NMU):*   Three groups of 63 female Wistar *rats* were treated with a single intravesicular dose of 0.15 ml of a saturated solution of NMU in saline.   Two weeks later, *ortho*-toluenesulphonamide (Monsanto Industrial Chemicals Co., USA;   pure) was administered at levels of 0, 0.08 mg/kg bw in the diet or 0.1% in the drinking-water for 2 years.   Survival was similar in all groups at 84 weeks.   No difference in overall tumour incidence was seen between control and test groups.   Neoplasia and hyperplasia of the bladder occurred in 27% and 35%, respectively, of rats in the NMU control group.   No statistical increase in bladder neoplasia or hyperplasia was observed in groups given NMU and *ortho*-toluenesulphonamide (Hooson *et al.*, 1980).

3.2   Other relevant biological data

(a)   Experimental systems

Toxic effects

Saccharin and its salts

The LD_{50} values for sodium saccharin by oral administration are: mice, 17.5 g/kg bw; random-bred rats, 17 g/kg bw;   Wistar rats, 14.2 g/kg bw (Taylor *et al.*, 1968); hamster, 8.7 and 7.4 g/kg bw, in males and females, respectively (Althoff *et al.*, 1975).   The LD_{50} by i.p. injection is: mice, 6.3 g/kg bw;   random-bred rats, 7.1 g/kg bw (Taylor *et al.*, 1968).

Addition of 0.5% sodium saccharin to the diet reduced the growth rate of rats over a 38-day period.   The feeding of 0.065 g/kg bw per day sodium saccharin to dogs for 11 months produced no toxic effect other than occasional stool softening (Taylor *et al.*, 1968).

Addition of 2% sodium saccharin to the diet of dogs for 16 weeks or of rats for 13 weeks had no noticeable toxic effects (Kennedy et al., 1976). Hamsters given 1.25% saccharin for 8 weeks in their drinking-water showed no toxic effects (Althoff et al., 1975). Administration of 1% sodium saccharin in drinking-water and/or 5% in food decreased weight gain and caused death in rats fed reduced food rations (Strouthes, 1978).

Administration to rats of 2 g/kg bw per day sodium saccharin in the drinking-water or of 4 g/kg bw per day in the diet reduced weight gain markedly; fluid intake was increased in the latter group and decreased in the former. The urinary pH of males of the first group rose above 7.0 after 27 weeks, and some animals showed marked crystalluria. These pH changes were reversible. The most important treatment-related findings were increased incidences of microcalculi and telangiectasia of the vasa recta in kidneys, of renal pelvic hyperplasia , of extramedullary haematopoiesis and of hepatic zonal necrosis. Hyperplasia of the bladder epithelium occurred earlier in animals of the second group (Chowaniec & Hicks, 1979).

In a six-generation experiment with Swiss mice receiving 0.2 or 0.5% saccharin (containing 0.5% ortho-toluenesulphonamide) in their diet, no effect on weight gain and no histopathological alterations due to treatment were found in long-term studies (21 months) performed with the 1st, 3rd and 6th generations (Kroes et al., 1977).

Saccharin is a competitive inhibitor of glucose-6-phosphatase in vitro (Lygre, 1974, 1976) and inhibits guanylate cyclase (Vesely & Levey, 1978). It also inhibited the induction of liver tryptophan oxygenase (Sabri et al., 1969).

Chronic feeding of 7.5% sodium saccharin in the diets of rats inhibited epithelial DNA synthesis in the urinary bladder (Lawson, 1978).

ortho-*Toluenesulphonamide*

The LD_{50} by oral administration in rats is about 2 g/kg bw (Schmähl, 1978).

Teratogenicity and embryotoxicity

No effects on reproduction were observed in 20 mice receiving 194 mg/kg bw saccharin daily for 180 days (Lehmann, 1929). Oral doses of up to 600 mg/kg bw per day saccharin or its sodium salt given over the total organogenesis phase have not been found to induce malformations or other embryotoxic effects in mice (Lorke, 1969), rats (Fritz & Hess, 1968; Lessel, 1971) or rabbits (Klotzsche, 1969; Lessel, 1971).

Feeding of male and female mice for 10 weeks with a diet containing 1% sodium sacc-harin, corresponding to a daily intake of about 2000 mg/kg bw, had no effect on their fer-tility when subsequently mated and caused no biologically important increase in pre-implan-tative or post-implantative losses (Lorke & Machemer, 1975).

Multigeneration experiments, including studies on reproductive capacity and perinatal development, and teratological studies, performed with Swiss mice receiving 0.2 or 0.5% saccharin in the diet revealed no pathological effects (Kroes et al., 1977).

Tanaka (1964) reported that saccharin is about 100 times more toxic to fetal than to adult mice; however, these data appear to contradict all other results. Serious doubts have been raised about the validity of Tanaka's data and his experimental approach (Lorke, 1969), and Tanaka et al. (1973) could not confirm his earlier findings.

. It was reported in an abstract that in a three-generation reproduction study with Charles River CD rats, average weaning weights were decreased compared with controls in litters from parents that received 5 or 7.5% sodium saccharin in the diet, but survival was not affected. Other reproductive indices showed scattered variations, but were not consistent over all generations (Taylor & Friedman, 1974).

It was reported in an abstract that no significant increase in fetal deaths, number of resorptions or drug-induced teratogenic effect was found in hamsters administered 10 and 100 g/day of calcium saccharin or a mixture of calcium saccharin and calcium cyclamate ('Sucaryl') during pregnancy. A decrease in litter size was seen in rats given the highest dose. No decrease in survival from birth to weaning was seen in either hamsters or rats (Adkins et al., 1972).

No evidence of a primary embryotoxic effect was seen in Wistar rats treated with 0.4% sodium saccharin [meeting the standards established in the Federal Republic of Germany (see section 1.4)] for 20 days after mating; histological examination revealed no ocular damage at term or at the age of 3 weeks. Impurities were not tested (Luckhaus & Machemer, 1978).

While the majority of investigators found no abnormalities in animals treated with saccharin during pregnancy, Lederer (1977) and Lederer & Pottier-Arnould (1973) reported morphological changes of the eye lens and increased embryonic mortality in offspring of pregnant Wistar rats fed 0.3 and 3% saccharin in the diet. Lederer (1977) concluded that the anomalies found were due to impurities in commercial saccharin synthesized by the Remsen-Fahlberg method, since the anomalies did not occur in animals treated with saccharin made by the Maumee procedure. The contaminating compounds of the saccharin produced by the Remsen-Fahlberg method, when tested separately, also induced ocular changes. ortho-Sulphobenzoic acid was most active when added to feed at a level of 0.1%; ortho-sulpha-moylbenzoic acid and ammonium-ortho-sulphobenzoic acid at dietary levels of 0.1% also increased the incidence of both ocular abnormalities and mortality over that seen in controls; and *ortho*-toluenesulphonamide was almost inactive. Lederer reported that a few ocular abnormalities also occurred in his controls [The possibility of histological artefacts has not been ruled out]. Lederer & Pottier-Arnould (1969) found an increased mortality in the off-spring of mice given 5% saccharin in their diet.

It was reported in an abstract that no toxicological changes were noted in dogs that received 0.5-1.5 g/kg bw per day of a 10:1 combination of sodium cyclamate:sodium saccharin [corresponding to daily doses of 45-140 mg/kg bw sodium saccharin] during pregnancy or in their offspring that received the same dose up to the age of one year (Fancher *et al.*, 1968).

Absorption, distribution, excretion and metabolism

Saccharin

^{14}C-Saccharin administered by i.v. infusion to 5 rhesus monkeys (4 μg/kg bw per min for 60 min) in the last trimester of pregnancy crossed the placenta rapidly and was distributed in all fetal tissues except the central nervous system. At the end of the infusion period, fetal blood levels were approximately 30% of maternal values. In contrast to the maternal organism, in which radioactivity decreased quickly after infusion ended, saccharin cleared very slowly from the fetal compartment, and 2 hours after termination of the infusion, fetal blood levels were higher than maternal ones. The slow rate of fetal clearance suggests that considerable accumulation might result from repetitive maternal ingestion. No data were available on the penetration of saccharin into the embryonic compartment during the organogenesis stage (Pitkin *et al.*, 1971a).

Saccharin was excreted rapidly unchanged by rhesus monkeys (Pitkin *et al.*, 1971b) and by guinea-pigs; about 70% was found in rat urine and the remainder in the faeces (Minegishi *et al.*, 1972). Although it is rapidly excreted by rats, some accumulates in the bladder; but after removal of saccharin from the diet, it is completely cleared within 3 days (Matthews *et al.*, 1973). Lethco & Wallace (1975) also found that the highest levels of radioactivity after administration of ^{14}C-labelled saccharin were in the kidney and bladder and that the metabolic profiles of dogs, rabbits, guinea-pigs and hamsters were similar.

Sodium ^{35}S-saccharin instilled into the bladder of male rats was absorbed into the plasma (Colburn, 1978).

The accumulation of saccharin by rat renal cortical tissue incubated *in vitro* was dependent upon oxygen and was reduced by metabolic inhibitors, suggesting that saccharin is eliminated by active tubular secretion (Goldstein *et al.*, 1978). Saccharin forms ion-pair complexes with bases such as quinine and ephedrine and facilitates the absorption of these bases from the rat rectum (Kakemi *et al.*, 1969).

In many studies on the metabolism of saccharin in several animal species, no metabolites have been detected. Byard & Golberg (1973) showed that 90% of ^{14}C-labelled saccharin was excreted unchanged by rats and monkeys of both sexes. Even after pretreatment with phenobarbitone or sodium saccharin no metabolites of saccharin were found. Ball et al. (1977) showed that it was not metabolized by liver microsomal preparations or by faecal homogenates taken from rats fed 1% saccharin in the diet for 2 years. No binding of saccharin to DNA of rat liver and urinary bladder was found 5 hours after oral administration of 372-390 mg/kg bw ^{35}S-saccharin (Lutz & Schlatter, 1977).

ortho-*Toluenesulphonamide and other impurities*

Of the more than 30 impurities that have been identified in commercial saccharin, data on metabolism are available for only a few. The rates at which 7 intragastrically administered impurities of saccharin [radiolabelled ortho-toluenesulphonamide, benz(d)isothiazoline-1,1-dioxide, 3-aminobenz(d)isothiazoline-1,1-dioxide, 5-chlorosaccharin, toluene-4-sulphonamide and 4-sulphamoylbenzoic acid] were eliminated in rats were similar. At doses ranging from 20-80 mg/kg bw, 80-95% of the impurities were recovered within 24 hours in urine and faeces; urinary metabolites of these impurities were identified (Ball et al., 1978; Renwick, 1978; Renwick & Williams, 1978; Renwick et al., 1978).

In female Wistar rats given single oral doses of 20, 125 or 200 mg/kg bw ^{14}C-ortho-toluenesulphonamide, 79, 58 and 36% of the activity were recovered in 24-hour urine samples; 24-48-hour elimination was 7, 14 and 33% of the dose, respectively. Within 7 days, 4.5, 5.9 and 7% of the activity was recovered from the faeces. The main metabolites in the urine were 2-sulphamoylbenzyl alcohol and its sulphate or glucuronic acid conjugates (80%), N-acetyltoluene-2-sulphonamide (6%), saccharin (3%) and 2-sulphamoylbenzoic acid (2%) (Renwick et al., 1978).

In a similar study, 50% of administered ortho- and para-toluenesulphonamides excreted in urine had been metabolized to ortho- and para-sulphamoylbenzoic acids, respectively (Minegishi et al., 1972).

Mutagenicity and other short-term tests

Saccharin

Saccharin of various degrees of purity was not found to be mutagenic in the Salmonella/microsome assay when the standard plate method was used (Ashby et al., 1978; McCann, 1977; Pool, 1978; Stoltz et al., 1977).

There is an isolated report that a pharmaceutical preparation of saccharin was weakly mutagenic to TA98 and TA100 strains when a modified plate procedure using reisolated strains of the standard *Salmonella* assay tester strains was followed; the urine of mice given 2.5 g/kg bw pure or impure saccharin orally was also reported to be mutagenic to reisolated strains of TA98 and TA100 with this modified protocol (Batzinger *et al.*, 1977).

Mutagenic effects of both purified and impure lots of sodium saccharin have been observed in mouse lymphoma L5178Y cells in the presence of liver homogenate in a dose range of 10-14 mg/ml. Increases in the frequency of trifluorothymidine-resistant mutants were extremely small, and no clear dose-response effect was obtained (Clive *et al.*, 1979).

A highly purified preparation of saccharin [synthesized by the Maumee process, provided by Dr R. Stoltz, Canada] caused a significant, dose-related increase in chromosome aberrations (breaks, gaps, translocations and ring formations) in Chinese hamster ovary (CHO) cells in the presence of liver homogenate (McCann, 1977). It was reported in an abstract that chromatid breaks and gaps were also induced in CHO-K1 cells treated with sodium saccharin (purity unspecified) (Yoshida *et al.*, 1978). Aberrations have been induced by saccharin and its sodium salt in other Chinese hamster cell lines (Abe & Sasaki, 1977; Ishidate & Odashima, 1977; Kristoffersson, 1972; Masubuchi *et al.*, 1978a).

I.p. injections of 4 g/kg bw sodium saccharin significantly increased chromosome breaks and gaps in bone-marrow cells of male mice (Masubuchi *et al.*, 1978a), but not in those of hamsters given 1.5 g/kg bw saccharin orally for 3 days (van Went-de Vries & Kragten, 1975); Leonard & Leonard (1979) obtained negative results with male C57Bl mice injected intraperitoneally with 4 g/kg bw sodium saccharin. No chromosome damage was detected in spermatogonia of Chinese hamsters given two doses of 5 g/kg bw sodium saccharin orally (Machemer & Lorke, 1975), or in spermatocytes of male C57Bl mice given 20 g saccharin/l drinking-water for 100 days (Leonard & Leonard, 1979).

Sister chromatid exchanges were induced by saccharin and its sodium salt in human (Wolff & Rodin, 1978) and hamster cells (Abe & Sasaki, 1977; Wolff & Rodin, 1978) *in vitro*.

Rao & Qureshi (1972) observed an increase in the number of dominant lethal mutations following administration to 20 male mice of 1.72% sodium saccharin in drinking-water for 30 days. Šrám & Zudová (1974) reported a dose-related increase in the incidence of dominant lethal mutations in mice, with a maximum frequency after 5 i.p. injections of 200 mg/kg bw sodium saccharin. In the same experiment, translocations and other aberrations in spermatocyte chromosomes were induced by this treatment. Masubuchi *et al.* (1978b) found a statistically significant increase in dominant lethal mutations within 2 weeks after treatment in mice given a single i.p. injection of 2 g/kg bw sodium saccharin; fertility of treated animals was low. Oral doses of 5 g/kg bw sodium saccharin given to NMRI mice for 5 days or of 20 g saccharin/l drinking-water given to C57Bl mice for 100 days had no effect on dominant lethality (Machemer & Lorke, 1973).

In several experiments testing saccharin in *Drosophila melanogaster*, no sex-linked recessive lethal mutations were induced (McCann, 1977; Samuel & Rao, 1972); however, the limit of sensitivity in the most extensive of these studies was detection of a 4-fold increase in the incidence of recessive lethal mutations (McCann, 1977). Some batches of commercial saccharin induced recessive lethal mutations in *Drosophila*, while others did not (Kramers, 1977), so that earlier positive results (Šrám & Weidenhofferová, 1969; Šrám & Zudová, 1972) may have been due to contaminants.

It was reported in an abstract that sodium saccharin caused a dose-related increase in unscheduled DNA synthesis in human fibroblasts treated *in vitro* (Ochi & Tonomura, 1978). There was no evidence of mitotic recombination in *Saccharomyces cerevisiae* D3 (McCann, 1977).

An impure sample used in the cancer bioassay of the Health Protection Branch of Canada (Arnold *et al.*, 1977, 1979) and purified samples of saccharin (provided by Dr R. Stoltz, Canada) (2 mg/ml) did not produce oncogenic transformation of C3H/10T½ mouse embryo fibroblasts *in vitro*. However, after treatment of the cells with a nontransforming initiating dose (0.1% μg/ml) of 3-methylcholanthrene, continuous treatment with either sample of saccharin (100 μg/ml) led to significant transformation. In this system saccharin was 1000-fold less active than the tumour promoter 12-*O*-tetradecanoyl-phorbol-13-acetate (Mondal *et al.*, 1978).

ortho-*Toluenesulphonamide and other impurities*

ortho-Toluenesulphonamide was not mutagenic in the *Salmonella*/microsome plate assay using strains TA98, TA100, TA1535, TA1537 and TA1538, with or without Arochlor 1254-induced rat liver 9000 x *g* supernatant. The doses used were up to 1 mg/plate (Jagannath & Brusick, 1978; Stoltz *et al.*, 1977) and 2.5 mg/plate (Ashby *et al.*, 1978). A similar study with negative results was reported by Poncelet *et al.* (1979). Wild *et al.* (1980) obtained a doubling of the mutation rate in TA98 at very high doses (up to 14 mg/plate) in the presence of Arochlor-induced rat-liver 9000 x *g* supernatant and only on a special medium other than the Vogel-Bonner-E-medium. A very similar effect was observed with *para*-toluenesulphonamide.

Impurities extracted with organic solvents from some lots of saccharin were active in tester strains TA98, TA1538 and TA100 (McCann, 1977; Stoltz *et al.*, 1977). *ortho*-Sulpho-benzoic acid and ammonium *ortho*-sulphobenzoic acid were not mutagenic in the standard tester strains of *Salmonella typhimurium*, with or without rat liver post-mitochondrial fraction (Poncelet *et al.*, 1979).

Doses of up to 1 mg/plate *ortho*-toluenesulphonamide did not induce gene conversion in *Saccharomyces cerevisiae* strain D4, with or without metabolic activation (Jagannath & Brusick, 1978).

Injection of 0.2 µl or feeding of 5 mM of *ortho*-toluenesulphonamide did not increase the incidence of sex-linked recessive lethal mutations in *Drosophila melanogaster* (Kramers, 1977); however, in a larger-scale study, Wild *et al.* (1980) found a statistically significant doubling of the frequency after 3 days' feeding of a 0.05% solution of *ortho*- or *para*-toluene-sulphonamide.

No increase in the number of breaks, gaps and other aberrations was seen in CHO-K1 cells after 24-hours' treatment with 0.9-400 µg/ml *ortho*-toluenesulphonamide (Masubuchi *et al.*, 1977, 1978c).

Concentrations of 0.025-2500 µg/ml *ortho*-toluenesulphonamide produced no morpho-logical transformation in BHK 21/Cl 13 cells (Ashby *et al.*, 1978). Oral and i.p. doses of up to 2 x 1 g/kg bw *ortho*- and *para*- toluenesulphonamide did not induce micronuclei in mouse bone-marrow cells (Wild *et al.*, 1980).

(b) Humans

Saccharin

Doses of more than 3 g saccharin per day cause some disturbances in digestion (Neumann, 1926). No metabolic disturbances were observed in subjects with diabetes mellitus administered 8 g saccharin (Pröls *et al.*, 1973). Allergic reactions to saccharin have been reported (Gordon, 1972; Miller *et al.*, 1974); and Fujita *et al.* (1965) reported 5 patients in whom oral administration of 0.1 g saccharin caused pruritis and oedematous papules on the trunk and limbs.

Saccharin diffuses into lymph, cerebrospinal fluid, saliva, tears and milk (Carlson *et al.*, 1923). About 90% of that present in plasma is bound to serum albumin (Ågren & Bäck, 1973).

In 3 volunteers, 85-92% of doses of 1 g [3-^{14}C]-saccharin administered orally for 21 days was excreted unchanged in the urine within 24 hours; no metabolites were found (Ball *et al.*, 1977). Within 48 hours, 92.3% of a dose of 500 mg ^{14}C-saccharin was excreted in the urine and 5.8% in the faeces (Byard *et al.*, 1974).

Stone *et al.* (1971) studied 975 women delivered of children who were not mentally retarded and women delivered of 247 mentally retarded children. They found that more mothers of children with Down's syndrome and other causes of mental retardation had used artificial sweeteners before and during pregnancy than had controls (Table 4).

Table 4. Mothers of mentally retarded and normal children who had used artificial sweeteners during pregnancy

	Year of delivery		
	1959-61	1962-64	1965-69
Mothers of mentally retarded children	14/79 (17.7%)	26/115 (22.6%)	19 53 (35.8%)
Mothers of normal children	9/78 (11.5%) not significant	35/242 (14.5%) $\chi^2=4.75$, P<0.05	141/655 (21.5%) $\chi^2=4.96$, P<0.05
Relative risk[1]	1.7	1.7	2.0

In addition, the study showed that users of artificial sweeteners had an increased incidence of other adverse outcomes of pregnancy: 'behavioural problems' (incidences - 5.4%, 10/ 185, in children of artificial sweetener users and 2.0%, 15/790, in children of non-users) and 'physical anomalies' (mainly deformities of the bones and joints of the hip, leg and foot; incidences - 4.8%, 9/185, in children of artificial sweetener users and 1.5%, 12/790, in children of non-users [P<0.01]) [Neither age, parity, smoking habits, the presence of diabetes mellitus nor socio-economic status were controlled for in the analysis, and no data were presented on how much artificial sweetener was used. The diverse effects found might argue against a direct effect of the artificial sweeteners, particularly in the absence of a prior expectation that exposure to such agents may cause such abnormalities. Further epidemiological data are needed before concluding that the use of artificial sweeteners in pregnancy is associated with fetal damage].

Kline *et al.* (1978) compared saccharin use in 545 women who had had spontaneous abortions (<28 weeks gestation) and that in 308 women delivering after 28 weeks. Cases were matched with controls within 2 years of age at last menstrual period. There were no statistically significant differences between cases and controls with respect to language spoken at interview, marital status, ethnic group or education level of patient or husband. Occupational level and mean income were slightly greater in cases, and controls more often reported welfare as the principal source of income [These last two factors were not controlled for in the analysis]. Age at last menstrual period, number of previous abortions, smoking and obesity were controlled for using a multiple logistic regression analysis, and diabetics and suspected diabetics were excluded. Saccharin was used by 30 cases (5.5%) and by 18 controls (5.8%) (relative risk, 0.94; 95% confidence interval, 0.5-1.8) [Information

[1] Calculated by the Working Group

on the intake of saccharin did not include use of presweetened drinks and food. No data were available on whether saccharin was used before or during pregnancy, or both, and no information on dose was presented. Most chromosomally abnormal conceptions are lost quite early in pregnancy (often before a women may even be aware that she is pregnant), and, as the authors point out, few women aborting for this reason will be included in a hospital series. This factor cannot be evaluated fully, since the gestational ages of the cases are not reported].

ortho-*Toluenesulphonamide*

Low oral doses of 0.2-0.4 mg/kg bw ^{14}C-*ortho*-toluenesulphonamide were excreted more slowly in humans than in rats, with about 50% of the activity being excreted in the urine within 24 hours and 80% within 48 hours. Less than 1% of the activity was found in faeces. The main urinary metabolites were 2-sulphamoylbenzyl alcohol and its sulphate and glucuronic acid conjugates (35%), saccharin (35%), 2-sulphamoylbenzoic acid (4%) and *N*-acetyltoluene-2-sulphonamide (2%) (Renwick *et al.*, 1978).

3.3 Case reports and epidemiological studies

See **Studies in Humans of Cancer in Relation to the Consumption of Artificial, Non-nutritive Sweetening Agents,** pp. 171-183.

4. Summary of Data Reported and Evaluation

4.1 Experimental data

Saccharin has been tested by oral administration in mice, rats and hamsters. In mice, saccharin produced no difference in tumour incidence between treated and control animals in one single and in one multigeneration study. Two further studies by oral administration in mice and three in rats were considered to be inadequate for evaluation. A study in hamsters by oral administration and one study in mice by skin application could not be evaluated. A study in mice by bladder insertion provided evidence for the induction of bladder carcinomas.

Sodium saccharin has been tested by oral administration in mice, rats and monkeys. One study in mice was inadequate for evaluation. One single-generation study in rats showed an increased incidence of bladder tumours in males; two further studies showed a few bladder tumours; one other study showed no difference in tumour incidence between treated and control animals; and two others were inadequate for evaluation. In three two-generation studies in rats, sodium saccharin produced a statistically significant increase in bladder tumours in F_1 males. Sodium saccharin has also been tested in mice by bladder insertion (implantation): it increased the incidence of bladder carcinomas. It has also been tested by oral administration in monkeys and by intraperitoneal administration in mice, but these experiments were considered to be inadequate for evaluation.

The combination of sodium saccharin with sodium cyclamate in a ratio of 1:10 has been tested by oral administration in a multigeneration experiment in mice and in three single -generation experiments in rats. In one study in rats, transitional-cell carcinomas in the bladder were produced in male animals given the highest dose; in a further study in rats and in the study in mice, there was no difference in tumour incidence between treated and control animals. The other study in rats was inadequate for evaluation.

In one study, female rats were administered sodium saccharin in the drinking-water or diet after receiving a single instillation into the bladder of a low dose of N-nitroso-N-methyl-urea (NMU): a high incidence of transitional-cell neoplasms of the bladder was found compared with animals that received NMU alone. Sodium saccharin was also tested in male rats pretreated with N-[4(5-nitro-2-furyl)-2-thiazolyl] formamide, resulting in an increased incidence of carcinomas of the bladder over that seen in rats given the latter compound alone.

ortho-Toluenesulphonamide was tested by oral administration in rats in a two-generation study: no increase in bladder tumour incidence was noted in animals of either generation. In one of two single-generation studies in rats, benign and malignant bladder tumours were found.

There is little evidence that saccharin itself induces point mutations. Dominant lethal effects and unscheduled DNA synthesis have been reported; and it causes sister chromatid exchanges and other chromosomal effects.

In the majority of the studies, no indication for a teratogenic effect of saccharin was found; impurities may be responsible for the occasional effects reported. There is no evidence that ortho-toluenesulphonamide is mutagenic, although impurities extracted from some lots of saccharin were mutagenic in the Salmonella/microsome test. In one in vitro test, saccharin was found to enhance the neoplastic transformation of fibroblasts treated with 3-methylcholanthrene.

4.2 Human data

Mortality from bladder cancer has been investigated in two studies by examination of time trends in the United States and in England and Wales. These have shown no marked increase in incidence or mortality from bladder cancer following a substantial increase over a few years in the use of cyclamates and saccharin, but such studies are too insensitive to exclude completely a carcinogenic effect.

In two studies of cancer mortality in patients with diabetes mellitus (who, as a group, have been shown to consume larger quantities of artificial sweeteners than the general population), lower mortality from cancer at all sites was observed as compared with the general population; there was no excess of bladder cancer in particular. In a further study, the frequency of the mention of diabetes mellitus in death certificates of persons who had died of bladder cancers was compared with that in those of controls who had died of other cancers (excluding the lung and pancreas); in the presence of diabetes mellitus, there was no increase in the risk of bladder cancer. As there are differences other than artificial sweetener use between diabetics and the general population, such studies cannot exclude a small carcinogenic effect of these sweeteners.

Seven case-control studies were considered by the Working Group. Only two of these studies examined confounding factors in detail. Of these two, one suggested that use of nine or more tablets of artificial sweeteners per day (or more than eight tablets of saccharin per day) was positively associated with risk for bladder cancer in men but not in women, although in these small groups the results may have been due to chance, to unsuspected confounding factors, or to residual effects of those confounding factors that were considered in the analysis and could be shown to reduce the magnitude of the association. The other study that considered confounding factors suggested that there was no effect of the use of artificial sweeteners on the incidence of bladder cancer; the observed relative risk was 1.0 (indicating no increase in risk), but a relative risk below 1.4 could not be excluded. The other five case-control studies also showed no association, although they were limited by some inadequacies in experimental design.

In six of the seven case-control studies, women with bladder cancer showed a tendency to consume less artificial sweeteners than female controls. This observation suggests that there is no association between use of artifical sweeteners and bladder cancer in women.

4.3 Evaluation [1]

Although a small increase in the risk of urinary bladder cancer in the general population or a larger increase in some individuals consuming very high doses of saccharin and cyclamates cannot be excluded, the epidemiological data provide no clear evidence that saccharin alone, or in combination with cyclamates, causes urinary bladder cancer. There are no epidemiological studies on a possible association between use of saccharin and cyclamates and cancer at other sites in humans.

There is *sufficient evidence* that saccharin alone, given at high doses, produces tumours of the urinary tract in male rats and can promote the action of known carcinogens in the bladder of rats of both sexes; and there is *limited evidence* of its carcinogenicity in mice. There is *limited evidence* that *ortho*-toluenesulphonamide is carcinogenic when given orally to rats; but the available data suggest that impurities at the levels normally found in commercial saccharin do not contribute to the carcinogenicity of saccharin.

[1] See footnote pp. 182-183

5. References

Abe, S. & Sasaki, M. (1977) Chromosome aberrations and sister chromatid exchanges in Chinese hamster cells exposed to various chemicals. *J. natl Cancer Inst., 58*. 1635-1641

Adkins, A., Hupp, E.W. & Gerdes, R.A. (1972) Biological activity of saccharins and cyclamates in golden hamsters (Abstract). *Texas J. Sci., 23,* 575

Ågren, A. & Bäck, T. (1973) Complex formation between macromolecules and drugs. VIII. Binding of saccharine, *N*-methyl saccharine, and the diuretic drugs hydroflumethiazide and bendroflumethiazide to human serum albumin. *Acta pharm. suecica, 10,* 223-228

Allen, M.J., Boyland, E., Dukes, C.E., Horning, E.S. & Watson, J.G. (1957) Cancer of the urinary bladder induced in mice with metabolites of aromatic amines and tryptophan. *Br. J. Cancer, 11,* 212-231

Althoff, J., Cardesa, A., Pour, P. & Shubik, P. (1975) A chronic study of artificial sweeteners in Syrian golden hamsters. *Cancer Lett., 1,* 21-24

Anon. (1963) Maumee moves closer to optimum process to make saccharin. *Chemical Engineering News*, 9 December, pp. 76-78

Anon. (1978) Rules issued on saccharin warning label. *FDA Consumer*, February, pp. 4-5

Arnold, D.L., Moodie, C.A., Stavrić, B., Stoltz, D.R., Grice, H.C. & Munro, I.C. (1977) Canadian saccharin study. *Science, 197,* 320

Arnold, D.L., Moodie, C.A., Grice, H.C., Charbonneau, S.M., Stavrić, B., Collins, B.T., McGuire, P.F. & Munro, I.C. (1980) Long term toxicity of *ortho*toluenesulfonamide and saccharin in the rat. *Toxicol. appl. Pharmacol., 52,* 113-152

Ashby, J., Styles, J.A., Anderson, D. & Paton, D. (1978) Saccharin: an epigenetic carcinogen/mutagen? *Food Cosmet. Toxicol., 16,* 95-103

Ball, L.M., Renwick, A.G. & Williams, R.T. (1977) The fate of [^{14}C] saccharin in man, rat and rabbit and of 2-sulphamoyl [^{14}C] benzoic acid in the rat. *Xenobiotica, 7,* 189-203

Ball, L.M., Williams, R.T. & Renwick, A.G. (1978) The fate of saccharin impurities. The excretion and metabolism of [^{14}C] toluene-4-sulphonamide and 4-sulphamoyl [^{14}C]-benzoic acid in the rat. *Xenobiotica, 8,* 183-190

Batzinger, R.P., Ou, S.-Y.L. & Bueding, E. (1977) Saccharin and other sweeteners: mutagenic properties. *Science, 198*, 944-946

Beck, K.M. (1969) *Sweeteners, nonnutritive.* In: Kirk, R.E. & Othmer, D.F., eds, *Encyclopedia of Chemical Technology,* 2nd ed., Vol. 19, New York, John Wiley & Sons,
pp. 593-607

Belcher, R., Bogdanski, S.L., Sheikh, R.A. & Townshend, A. (1976) Determination of
saccharin in soft drinks by molecular emission cavity analysis. *Analyst, 101*, 562-565

Bio-Research Consultants, Inc. (1973) *Studies on Saccharin and Cyclamates,* Final Report,
Contract NIH-NCI-E-68-1311, Cambridge, MA, National Institutes of Health, Bethesda,
MD

Bryan, G.T., Ertürk, E. & Yoshida, O. (1970) Production of urinary bladder carcinomas in
mice by sodium saccharin. *Science, 168*, 1238-1240

Bundesminister der Justiz, ed. (1979) *Bundesgesetzblatt,* 4. Anlage 2, liste 12, Bonn,
Bundersanzeiger Verlagsges. mbH, pp. 82-83

Byard, J.L. & Golberg, L. (1973) The metabolism of saccharin in laboratory animals.
Food Cosmet. Toxicol., 11, 391-402

Byard, J.L., McChesney, E.W., Golberg, L. & Coulston, F. (1974) Excretion and metabolism
of saccharin in man. II. Studies with ^{14}C-labelled and unlabelled saccharin. *Food
Cosmet. Toxicol., 12*, 175-184

Canadian Health & Welfare Department (1977) Canadian position on saccharin. *News
Release 1977-40*, 9 March, Ottawa

Carlson, A.J., Eldridge, C.J., Martin, H.P. & Foran, F.L. (1923) Studies on the physiological action of saccharin. *J. Metab. Res., 3*, 451-477

Chowaniec, J. & Hicks, R.M. (1979) Response of the rat to saccharin with particular refer-
ence to the urinary bladder. *Br. J. Cancer, 39,* 355-375

Clive, D. Johnson, K.O., Spector, J.F.S., Batson, A.G. & Brown, M.M.M. (1979) Validation
and characterization of the L5178Y/TK[+/-] mouse lymphoma mutagen assay system.
Mutat. Res., 59, 61-108

Cohen, S.M., Arai, M., Jacobs, J.B. & Friedell, G.H. (1979) Promoting effect of saccharin and DL-tryptophan in urinary bladder carcinogenesis. *Cancer Res., 39*, 1207-1217

Colburn, W.A. (1978) Absorption of saccharin from rat urinary bladder. *J. pharm. Sci., 67*, 1493

Commission of the European Communities (1978) Commission recommendation of 29 March 1978 to the member states on the use of saccharin as a food ingredient and for sale as such in tablet form to the final consumer. *J. off. Communautés eur., L. 103*, 32

Coulston, F., McChesney, E.W. & Golberg, L. (1975) Long-term administration of artificial sweeteners to the rhesus monkey *(M. mulatta). Food Cosmet. Toxicol., 13*, 297-302

Crammer, B. & Ikan, R. (1977) Properties and syntheses of sweetening agents. *Chem. Soc. Rev., 6*, 431-453

Crampton, R.F. (1975) *The questions of benefits and risks.* In: *Sweeteners, Issues and Uncertainties*, Academy Forum, 4, Washington DC, National Academy of Sciences, pp. 127-132

Eng, M.-Y., Calayan, C. & Talmage, J.M. (1977) Determination of sodium saccharin in chewing gum by high pressure liquid chromatography. *J. Food Sci., 42*, 1060-1061

Ershoff, B. H. & Bajwa, G.S. (1974) Inhibitory effect of sodium cyclamate and sodium saccharin on tumor induction by 2-acetylaminofluorene in rats. *Proc. Soc. exp. Biol. (N.Y.), 145*, 1293-1297

Fancher, O.E., Palazzolo, R.J., Blockus, L., Weinberg, M.S. & Calandra, J.C. (1968) Chronic studies with sodium saccharin and sodium cyclamate in dogs (Abstract no. 15). *Toxicol. appl. Pharmacol., 12*, 291

Fitzhugh, O.G., Nelson, A.A. & Frawley, J.P. (1951) A comparison of the chronic toxicities of synthetic sweetening agents. *J. Am. pharm. Assoc., 40*, 583-586

Fritz, H. & Hess, R. (1968) Prenatal development in the rat following the administration of cyclamate, saccharin and sucrose. *Experientia, 24*, 1140-1141

Fujita, H., Kobayasi, T., Asagami, C., Iwao, E., Oda, Y. & Mori, T. (1965) Five cases which showed diffuse erythema and edematous papules, possibly caused by saccharin (Jpn.). *Acta dermatol. (Kyoto), 60*, 303-308

Furuya, T., Kawamata, K., Kaneko, T., Uchida, O., Horiuchi, S. & Ikeda, Y. (1975) Long-term toxicity study of sodium cyclamate and saccharin sodium in rats (Abstract). *Jpn. J. Pharmacol., 25*, 55P-56P

Goldstein, R.S., Hook, J.B. & Bond, J.T. (1978) Renal tubular transport of saccharin. *J. Pharmacol. exp. Ther., 204*, 690-695

Gordon, H.H. (1972) Allergic reactions to saccharin. *Am. J. Obstet. Gynecol., 113*, 1145

Grasselli, J.G., ed. (1973) *CRC Atlas of Spectral Data and Physical Constants for Organic Compounds,* Cleveland, OH, Chemical Rubber Co., p. B-969

Hartvig, R., Gyllenhaal, O. & Hammarlund, M. (1978) Determination of saccharin in urine by electron-capture gas chromatography after extractive methylation. *J. Chromatogr., 151,* 232-236

Hawley, G., ed. (1977) *The Condensed Chemical Dictionary*, 9th ed., New York, Van Nostrand-Rheinhold, p. 869

Hicks, R.M., Chowaniec, J. & Wakefield, J.StJ. (1978) *Experimental induction of bladder tumors by a two-stage system.* In: Slaga, T.J., Sivak, A. & Boutwell, R.K., eds, *Carcinogenesis*, Vol. 2, *Mechanisms of Tumor Promotion and Cocarcinogenesis,* New York, Raven Press, pp. 475-489

Homburger, F. (1978) *Negative lifetime carcinogen studies in rats and mice fed 50,000 ppm saccharin.* In: Galli, C.L., Paoletti, R. & Vettorazzi, G., eds, *Chemical Toxicology of Food*, Amsterdam, Elsevier/North-Holland Biomedical Press, pp. 359-373

Hooson, J., Hicks, R.M., Grasso, P. & Chowaniec, J. (1980) *ortho*-Toluene sulphonamide and saccharin in the promotion of bladder cancer in the rat. *Br. J. Cancer* (in press)

Hussein, M.M., Jacin, H. & Rodriguez, F.B. (1976) Quantitative determination of saccharin in food products by ultraviolet spectrometry. *J. agric. Food Chem., 24,* 36-40

IARC (1979) *Information Bulletin on the Survey of Chemicals Being Tested for Carcinogenicity,* No. 8, Lyon, pp. 90, 183, 300, 460

Ishidate, M., Jr & Odashima, S. (1977) Chromosome tests with 134 compounds on Chinese hamster cells *in vitro* - a screening for chemical carcinogens. *Mutat. Res., 48,* 337-354

Jacin, H, (1975) The quantitative determination of *ortho*-toluene sulfonamide (*o*-TS) in saccharin by U.V. spectrophotometry and by gas chromatography. *Dtsch. Lebensmittel-Rundschau, 71,* 428-429

Jagannath, D.R. & Brusick, D. (1978) *Mutagenicity Evaluation of ortho-Toluenesulphoneamide in the Ames* Salmonella/*Microsome Plate Test,* Final Report, submitted to AKZO, Arnhem, The Netherlands by Litton Bionetics Inc., Kensington, MD

Janiak, R.A., Damon, H.H. & Mohr, T.C. (1978) Determination of orthotoluenesulfonamide (OTS) in soluble saccharin. *J. agric. Food Chem., 26*, 710-711

Kakemi, K., Sezaki, H., Muranishi, S. & Tsujimura, Y. (1969) Absorption and excretion of drugs. XL. Enhancement of the rectal absorption of pharmaceutical amines with lauryl sulfate and saccharinate anions. *Chem. pharm. Bull., 17*, 1641-1650

Kennedy, G.L., Jr, Fancher, O.E. & Calandra, J.C. (1976) Subacute toxicity studies with sodium saccharin and two hydrolytic derivatives. *Toxicology, 6*, 133-138

Kline, J., Stein, Z.A., Susser, M. & Warburton, D. (1978) Spontaneous abortion and the use of sugar substitutes (saccharin). *Am. J. Obstet. Gynecol., 130*, 708-711

Klotzsche, C. (1969) The teratogenic and embryotoxic effect of cyclamate, saccharin and sucrose (Ger.). *Arzneimittel-Forsch., 19*, 925-928

Kramers, P.G.N. (1977) Mutagenicity of saccharin in *Drosophila*: the possible role of contaminants. *Mutat. Res., 56*, 163-167

Kristoffersson, U. (1972) The effect of cyclamate and saccharin on the chromosomes of a Chinese hamster cell line. *Hereditas, 70*, 271-282

Kroes, R., Peters, P.W.J., Berkvens, J.M., Verschuuren, H.G., De Vries, T. & van Esch, G.J. (1977) Long term toxicity and reproduction study (including a teratogenicity study) with cyclamate, saccharin and cyclohexylamine. *Toxicology, 8*, 285-300

Lawson, T.A. (1978) *Replication and permeability in the animal model.* In: Guggenheim, B., ed., *Health and Sugar Substitutes*, Basel, Karger, pp. 48-53

Lederer, J. (1977) Saccharin, its impurities and their teratogenic effect (Fr.). *Louvain Med., 96*, 495-501

Lederer, J. & Pottier-Arnould, A.M. (1969) Toxicity of sodium cyclamate and saccharin for the offspring of pregnant mice (Fr.). *Diabète, 17*, 103-106

Lederer, J. & Pottier-Arnould, A.M. (1973) Influence of saccharin on the development of the embryo in the gestating rat (Fr.). *Diabète, 21*, 13-16

Lehmann, K.B. (1929) Feeding study with and without saccharin on mice pairs and search for the minimal toxic effect (Ger.). *Arch. Hyg., 101*, 39-47

Leonard, A. & Leonard, E.D. (1979) Mutagenicity test with saccharin in the male mouse. *J. environ. Pahtol. Toxicol., 2*, 1047-1053

Lessel, B. (1971) *Carcinogenic and teratogenic aspects of saccharin.* In: *SOS/70 Proceedings of the Third International Congress of Food Science and Technology, Washington DC, 1970,* Chicago, IL,Institute of Food Technologists, pp. 764-770

Lethco, E.J. & Wallace, W.C. (1975) The metabolism of saccharin in animals. *Toxicology, 3,* 287-300

Lorke, D. (1969) Studies on the embryotoxic and teratogenic effects of cyclamate and saccharin in the mouse (Ger.). *Arzneimittel-Forsch., 19,* 920-922

Lorke, D. & Machemer, L. (1975) The effect of several weeks' treatment of male and female mice with saccharin, cyclamate or cyclohexylamine sulphate on fertility and dominant lethal effects (Ger.). *Humangenetik, 26,* 199-205

Luckhaus, G. & Machemer, L. (1978) Histological examination of perinatal eye development in the rat after ingestion of sodium cyclamate and sodium saccharin during pregnancy. *Food Cosmet. Toxicol., 16,* 7-11

Lutz, W.K. & Schlatter, C. (1977) Saccharin does not bind to DNA of liver or bladder in the rat. *Chem.-biol. Interactions, 19,* 253-257

Lygre, D.G. (1974) The inhibition by saccharin and cyclamate of phosphotransferase and phosphohydrolase activities of glucose-6-phosphatase. *Biochim. biophys. Acta, 341,* 291-297

Lygre, D.G. (1976) Inhibition by saccharin of glucose-6-phosphatase: effects of alloxan *in vivo* and deoxycholate *in vitro. Can. J. Biochem., 54,* 587-590

Machemer, L. & Lorke, D. (1973) Dominant lethal test in the mouse for mutagenic effects of saccharine. *Humangenetik, 19,* 193-198

Machemer, L. & Lorke, D. (1975) Method for testing mutagenic effects of chemicals on spermatogonia of the Chinese hamster. Results obtained with cyclophosphamide, saccharin, and cyclamate. *Arzneimittel-Forsch., 25,* 1889-1896

Masubuchi, M., Nawai, S., Hiraga, K. & Hirokado, M. (1977) Lack of the cytogenetic effects of saccharin and its impurities on CHO-K1 cells (Jpn.). *Ann. Rep. Tokyo Metr. Res. Lab. P.H., 28,* 159-161

Masubuchi, M., Yoshida, S., Hiraga, K. & Nawai, S. (1978a) The mutagenicity of sodium saccharin (S-Na). II. Cytogenetic studies (Abstract no. 18). *Mutat. Res., 54,* 219

Masubuchi, M., Takahashi, A., Takahashi, O., Yoshida, S., Ando, H., Kudo, K. & Hiraga, K. (1978b) The mutagenicity of sodium saccharin (S-Na). I. Dominant-lethal test (Abstract no. 17). *Mutat. Res., 54*, 218-219

Masubuchi, M., Nawai, S., Hirokado, M. & Hiraga, K. (1978c) Lack of the cytogenetic effects of saccharin impurities on CHO-K1 cells (Abstract no. 13). *Mutat. Res., 54*, 242-243

Matthews, H.B., Fields, M. & Fishbein, L. (1973) Saccharin: distribution and excretion of a limited dose in the rat. *J. agric. Food Chem., 21*, 916-919

McCann, J. (1977) *Short-term tests (Appendix II).* In: *Cancer Testing Technology and Saccharin*, Washington DC, Office of Technology Assessment, Congress of the United States, pp. 91-108

McChesney, E.W., Coulston, F. & Benitz, K.-F. (1977) Six-year study of saccharin in rhesus monkeys (Abstract no. 79). *Toxicol. appl. Pharmacol., 41*, 164

Miller, R., White, L.W. & Schwartz, H.J. (1974) A case of episodic urticaria due to saccharin ingestion. *J. Allerg. clin. Immunol., 53*, 240-242

Minegishi, K.-I., Asahina, M. & Yamaha, T. (1972) The metabolism of saccharin and the related compounds in rats and guinea pigs. *Chem. pharm. Bull., 20*, 1351-1356

Mockute, D. & Bernotiene, G. (1976) Determination of organic additives and their reaction products in electrolytes during metal electroplating. 5. Determination of benzamide, *o*-toluylamide, *o*-toluenesulfonamide, saccharin, phthalimidine, and phthalimide in nickel plating electrolytes when all are present (Russ.). *Liet. TSR Mokslu Akad. Darb., Ser. B, 3*, 87-90 [*Chem. Abstr., 86,* 65144v]

Mohr, U., Green, U., Althoff, J. & Schneider, P. (1978) *Syncarcinogenic action of saccharin and sodium-cyclamate in the induction of bladder tumours in MNU-pretreated rats.* In: Guggenheim, B., ed., *Health and Sugar Substitutes*, Basel, Karger, pp. 64-69

Mondal, S., Brankow, D.W. & Heidelberger, C. (1978) Enhancement of oncogenesis in C3H/10T½ mouse embryo cell cultures by saccharin. *Science, 201*, 1141-1142

Monsanto Industrial Chemicals Co. (undated) *Santicizer®9, Solid Processing Aid and Reactive Plasticizer*, Technical Bulletin IC/PL-9, Newport Beach, CA

Munro, I.C., Moodie, C.A., Krewski, D. & Grice, H.C. (1975) A carcinogenicity study of commercial saccharin in the rat. *Toxicol. appl. Pharmacol., 32*, 513-526

National Formulary Board (1970) *National Formulary XIII*, 13th ed., Washington DC, American Pharmaceutical Association, pp. 120-121, 644-645

National Formulary Board (1975) *National Formulary XIV*, 14th ed., Washington DC, American Pharmaceutical Association, pp. 642-645

National Institute of Hygienic Sciences (1973) *Chronic Toxicity Study of Sodium Saccharin: 21 Months Feeding in Mice*, Tokyo, Japan

National Research Council (1972) *Food Chemicals Codex*, 2nd ed., Washington DC, National Academy of Sciences, pp. 706-707, 764-765

National Research Council (1974) *Food Chemicals Codex*, 2nd ed., 1st Supplement, Washington DC, National Academy of Sciences, pp. 49, 56-58

National Research Council/National Academy of Sciences (1978) *Saccharin: Technical Assessment of Risks and Benefits*, Report No. 1, Committee for a Study on Saccharin and Food Safety Policy, Washington DC, Assembly of Life Sciences/Institute of Medicine

Neumann, R.O. (1926) Is the utilization of food protein influenced by saccharin? (Ger.) *Arch. Hyg., 96*, 265-276

Ochi, H. & Tonomura, A. (1978) Presence of unscheduled DNA synthesis in cultured human cells after treatment with sodium saccharin (Abstract no. 26). *Mutat. Res., 54*, 224

Oser, B.L., Carson, S., Cox, G.E., Vogin, E.E. & Sternberg, S.S. (1975) Chronic toxicity study of cyclamate:saccharin (10:1) in rats. *Toxicology, 4*, 315-330

Pitkin, R.M., Reynolds, W.A., Filer, L.J., Jr & Kling, T.G. (1971a) Placental transmission and fetal distribution of saccharin. *Am. J. Obstet. Gynecol., 111*, 280-286

Pitkin, R.M., Andersen, D.W., Reynolds, W.A. & Filer, L.J., Jr (1971b) Saccharin metabolism in *Macaca mulatta*. *Proc. Soc. exp. Biol. (N.Y.), 137*, 803-806

Poncelet, F., Roberfroid, M., Mercier, M. & Lederer, J. (1979) Absence of mutagenic activity in *Salmonella typhimurium* of some impurities found in saccharin. *Food Cosmet. Toxicol., 17*, 229-231

Pool, B. (1978) Non-mutagenicity of saccharin. *Toxicology, 11*, 95-97

Price, J.M., Biava, C.G., Oser, B.L., Vogin, E.E., Steinfeld, J. & Ley H.L. (1970) Bladder tumors in rats fed cyclohexylamine or high doses of a mixture of cyclamate and sodium. *Science, 167*, 1131-1132

Pröls, H., Haslbeck, M. & Mehnert, H. (1973) Studies on the effect of high doses of saccharin on the metabolism of diabetics (Ger.). *Dtsch. med. Wschr., 98*, 1901-1904

Rao, M.S., & Qureshi, A.B. (1972) Induction of dominant lethals in mice by sodium saccharin. *Indian J. med. Res., 60*, 599-603

Ratchik, E.M., & Viswanathan, V. (1975) GLC determination of saccharin in pharmaceutical products. *J. pharm. Sci., 64*, 133-135

Remsen, I. & Fahlberg, C. (1879) On the oxidation of substitution products of aromatic hydrocarbons. IV. On the oxidation of orthotoluenesulphamide. *J. Am. chem. Soc., 1*, 426-438

Renwick, A.G. (1978) The fate of saccharin impurities: the metabolism and excretion of 3-amino[3-^{14}C]benz[*d*]isothiazole-1,1-dioxide and 5-chlorosaccharin in the rat. *Xenobiotica, 8*, 487-494

Renwick, A.G. & Williams, R.T. (1978) The fate of saccharin impurities: the excretion and metabolism of [3-^{14}C]benz[*d*]isothiazoline-1,1-dioxide (BIT) in man and rat. *Xenobiotica, 8*, 475-486

Renwick, A.G., Ball, L.M., Corina, D.L. & Williams, R.T. (1978) The fate of saccharin impurities: the excretion and metabolism of toluene-2-sulphonamide in man and rat. *Xenobiotica, 8*, 461-474

Riggin, R.M., Kinzer, G.W., Margard, W.L., Mondron, P.J., Girod, F.T. & Birts, M.A. (1978) *Identification, Development of Methods for Analysis and Mutagenicity Testing of Impurities in Sodium Saccharin*, Columbus, OH, Battelle Columbus Laboratories

Roe, F.J.C., Levy, L.S. & Carter, R.L. (1970) Feeding studies on sodium cyclamate, saccharin and sucrose for carcinogenic and tumour-promoting activity. *Food Cosmet. Toxicol., 8*, 135-145

Sabri, M.I., Sharma, S.K. & Krishna Murti, C.R. (1969) Growth inhibitory action of saccharin and cyclamate on rats receiving a poor rice diet. *Br. J. Nutr., 23*, 505-509

Salaman, M.H. & Roe, F.J.C. (1956) Further tests for tumour-inititating activity: *N,N*-di-(2-chloroethyl)-*p*-aminophenylbutyric acid (CB1348) as an initiator of skin tumour formation in the mouse. *Br. J. Cancer, 10*, 363-378

Samuel, B.C. & Rao, M.S. (1972) Induction in *D. melanogaster* with *o*-sulphobenzoic imide (saccharin). *Drosophila Inform. Serv., 48*, 47

Schmähl, D. (1973) Lack of carcinogenic effect of cyclamate, cyclohexylamine and saccharin in rats (Ger.). *Arzneimittel-Forsch., 23*, 1466-1470

Schmähl, D. (1978) Experiments on the carcinogenic effect of ortho-toluol-sulfonamid (OTS). *Z. Krebsforsch., 91*, 19-22

The Sherwin-Williams Company (1977a) *Sodium Saccharin - Non-Nutritive Sweetener*, Technical Data Sheet 1, Chemicals Division, Cleveland, OH

The Sherwin-Williams Company (1977b) *Products Directory*, Technical Bulletin 741, Chemicals Division, Cleveland, OH, p. 3

The Sherwin-Williams Company (1978a) *Saccharin Insoluble Powder FCC - Non-Nutritive Sweetener*, Technical Data Sheet 2, Chemicals Division, Cleveland, OH

The Sherwin-Williams Company (1978b) *Sodium Saccharin Pelletized - Non-Nutritive Sweetener*, Technical Data Sheet 3, Chemicals Division, Cleveland OH

Sieber, S.M. & Adamson, R.H. (1978) *Long-term studies on the potential carcinogenicity of artificial sweeteners in non-human primates.* In: Guggenheim, B., ed., *Health and Sugar Substitutes*, Basel, Karger, pp. 266-271

Simko, J.P., Jr (1977) *Analysis of toothpastes.* In: Senzel, A.J., ed., *Newburger's Manual of Cosmetic Analysis*, 2nd ed., Washington DC, Association of Official Analytical Chemists, pp. 141-146

Smyly, D.A., Woodward, B.B. & Conrad, E.C. (1976) Determination of saccharin, sodium benzoate, and caffeine in beverages by reverse phase high-pressure liquid chromatography. *J. Assoc. off. anal. Chem., 59*, 14-19

Šrám, R.J. & Weidenhofferová, H. (1969) Mutagenic activity of saccharin. *Drosophila Inform. Serv., 44*, 120

Šrám, R.J., & Zudová, Z. (1972) Mutagenic activity of saccharin (Abstract no. 19), *EMS Newsl., 6*, 25

Šram, R.J. & Zudová, Z. (1974) Mutagenicity studies of saccharin in mice. *Bull. environ. Contam. Toxicol., 12*, 186-192

Stavrić, B., Lacombe, R., Watson, J.R. & Munro, I.C. (1974) Isolation, identification, and quantitation of *o*-toluenesulfonamide, a major impurity in commercial saccharins. *J. Assoc. off. anal. Chem., 57*, 678-681

Stavrić, B., Klassen, R. & By, A.W. (1976) Impurities in commercial saccharin. I. Impurities soluble in organic solvents. *J. Assoc. off. anal. Chem., 59*, 1051-1058

Stoltz, D.R., Stavrić, B., Klassen, R., Bendall, R.D. & Craig, J. (1977) The mutagenicity of saccharin impurities. I. Detection of mutagenic activity. *J. environ. Pathol. Toxicol., 1*, 139-146

Stone, D., Matalka, E. & Pulaski, B. (1971) Do artificial sweeteners ingested in pregnancy affect the offspring? *Nature, 231*, 53

Stoner, G.D., Shimkin, M.B., Kniazeff, A.J., Weisburger, J.H., Weisburger, E.K. & Gori, G.B. (1973) Test for carcinogenicity of food additives and chemotherapeutic agents by the pulmonary tumor response in strain A mice. *Cancer Res., 33*, 3069-3085

Strouthes, A. (1978) Mortality and the concurrent ingestion of food and saccharin in rats. *Physiol. Psychol., 6*, 89-92

Szinai, S.S. & Roy, T.A. (1976) Pyrolysis GLC identification of food and drug ingredients. I. Saccharin. *J. chromatogr. Sci., 14*, 327-330

Tanaka, A., Nose, N., Suzuki, T., Kobayashi, S. & Watanabe, A. (1977) Determination of saccharin in soft drinks by a spectrophotometric method. *Analyst, 102*, 367-370

Tanaka, R. (1964) LD_{50} of the saccharin or cyclamate for mice embryo in the 7th day of pregnancy (fetal median lethal dose: FLD_{50}). *J. Iwate med. Assoc., 16*, 330-337

Tanaka, S., Kawashima, K., Nakaura, S., Nagao, S., Kuwamura, T. & Omori, Y. (1973) Studies on the teratogenicity of food additives. I. Effects of saccharin sodium on the development of rats and mice. *J. Food Hyg. Soc., 14*, 371-379

Taylor, J.D., Richards, R.K., Wiegand, R.G. & Weinberg, M.S. (1968) Toxicological studies with sodium cyclamate and saccharin. *Food Cosmet. Toxicol., 6*, 313-327

Taylor, J.M. & Friedman, L. (1974) Combined chronic feeding and three-generation reproduction study of sodium saccharin in the rat (Abstract no. 200). *Toxicol appl. Pharmacol., 29*, 154

Tenenbaum, M. & Martin, G.E. (1977) High pressure liquid chromatographic determination of saccharin in alcoholic products. *J. Assoc. off. anal. Chem., 60*, 1321-1323

Tisdel, M.O., Nees, P.O., Harris, D.L. & Derse, P.H. (1974) *Long-term feeding of saccharin in rats.* In: Inglett, G.E., ed, *Symposium: Sweeteners,* Westport, CN, Avi Publishing Co., pp. 145-158

Ulland, B., Weisburger, E.K. & Weisburger, J.H. (1973) Chronic toxicity and carcinogenicity of industrial chemicals and pesticides (Abstract no. 19). *Toxicol. appl. Pharmacol., 25,* 446

US Department of Commerce (1978) *US Imports for Consumption and General Imports,* FT 246/December 1977, Bureau of the Census, Washington DC, US Government Printing Office, p. 1211

US Department of Health, Education, & Welfare (1973a) *Subacute and Chronic Toxicity, and Carcinogenicity of Sodium Saccharin,* Final Report, Project P-169-170, Division of Pathology, Washington DC, Food & Drug Administration

US Department of Health, Education, & Welfare (1973b) *Histopathologic Evaluation of Tissues from Rats following Continuous Dietary Intake of Sodium Saccharin and Calcium Cyclamate for a Maximum Period of Two Years,* Project P-169-170, Division of Pathology, Washington DC, Food & Drug Administration

US Food & Drug Administration (1977a) Food additives permitted in food for human consumption or in contact with food on an interim basis pending additional study. *Fed. Regist., 42,* 1461-1462

US Food & Drug Administration (1977b) Food additives: saccharin and its salts. *Fed. Regist., 42,* 1486-1487

US Food & Drug Administration (1977c) Saccharin and its salts: proposed rule making. *Fed. Regist., 42,* 19996-20010

US Food & Drug Administration (1978) Saccharin notice. *US Code Fed. Regul.,* Title 21, parts 101.11, 175.105, 180.37

US International Trade Commission (1976a) *Synthetic Organic Chemicals, US Production and Sales, 1974,* USITC Publication 776, Washington DC, US Government Printing Office, p. 120

US International Trade Commission (1976b) *Imports of Benzenoid Chemicals and Products, 1974,* USITC Publication 762, Washington DC, US Government Printing Office, p. 98

US International Trade Commission (1977a) *Saccharin from Japan and the Republic of Korea,* USITC Publication 846, Washington DC, US Government Printing Office, pp. A-4, A-7, A-42 - A-45

US International Trade Commission (1977b) *Synthetic Organic Chemicals, US Production and Sales, 1975,* USITC Publication 804, Washington DC, US Government Printing Office, p. 42

US International Trade Commission (1978a) *Synthetic Organic Chemicals, US Production and Sales, 1977*, USITC Publication 920, Washington DC, US Government Printing Office, pp. 200, 266

US International Trade Commission (1978b) *Imports of Benzenoid Chemicals and Products, 1977*, USITC Publication 900, Washington DC, US Government Printing Office, p. 94

US Pharmacopeial Convention, Inc. (1975) *The US Pharmacopeia*, 19th rev., Rockville, MD, pp. 568-569

US Tariff Commission (1922) *Census of Dyes and other Synthetic Organic Chemicals, 1921*, Tariff Information Series No. 26, Washington DC, US Government Printing Office, p. 25

US Tariff Commission (1940) *Synthetic Organic Chemicals, US Production and Sales, 1939*, Report No. 140, Second Series, Washington DC, US Government Printing Office, p. 48

US Tariff Commission (1954) *Synthetic Organic Chemicals, US Production and Sales, 1953*, Report No. 194, Second Series, Washington DC, US Government Printing Office, p. 114

US Tariff Commission (1974) *Imports of Benzenoid Chemicals and Products, 1973*, TC Publication 688, Washington DC, US Government Printing Office, p. 94

Vesely, D.L. & Levey, G.S. (1978) Saccharin inhibits guanylate cyclase activity: possible relationship to carcinogenesis. *Biochem. biophys. Res. Commun., 81*, 1384-1389

Wade, A., ed.(1977) *Martindale, The Extra Pharmacopoeia*, 27th ed., London, The Pharmaceutical Press, pp. 612-613

Weast, R.C., ed. (1977) *CRC Handbook of Chemistry and Physics*, 58th ed., Cleveland, OH, Chemical Rubber Co., pp. C-529, C-610, C-685

van Went-de Vries, G.F. & Kragten, M.C.T. (1975) Saccharin: lack of chromosome-damaging activity in Chinese hamsters *in vivo. Food Cosmet. Toxicol., 13*, 177-183

WHO (1976) Specifications for the identity and purity of some food colours, flavour en-hancers, thickening agents, and certain food additives. *WHO Food Addit. Ser., No. 7*, pp. 203-205, 211-216

WHO (1978) Evaluation of certain food additives. Twenty-first report of the Joint FAO/ WHO Expert Committee on Food Additives. *WHO tech. Rep. Ser., No. 617*, p. 25

Wild, D., Eckhardt, K., Gocke, E. & Kling, M.-T (1980) *Comparative results of short-term in vitro and in vivo mutagenicity tests obtained with selected environmental chemicals.* In: Norpoth, K. & Garner, R.C., eds, *Short-Term Mutagenicity Test Systems for Detecting Carcinogens,* Berlin, Springer (in press)

Windholz, M., ed (1976) *The Merck Index,* 9th ed., Rahway, NJ, Merck & Co., p. 1077

Wolff, S. & Rodin, B. (1978) Saccharin-induced sister chromatid exchanges in Chinese hamster and human cells. *Science, 200,* 543-545

Yamada, J. (1975) Artificial sweeteners. *Jpn chem. Rev.,* p. 68

Yoshida, S.M., Masubuchi, M. & Hiraga, K. (1978) Induced chromosome aberrations by artificial sweeteners in CHO-K1 cells (Abstract no. 45). *Mutat. Res., 54,* 262

STUDIES IN HUMANS OF CANCER IN RELATION TO THE CONSUMPTION OF ARTIFICIAL, NON-NUTRITIVE SWEETENING AGENTS

A general discussion of the use of epidemiological studies for establishing carcinogenicity is presented in the preamble to this volume, p. 16. The epidemiological data relating to cyclamates are not adequately separated from those relating to saccharin, and persons taking artificial sweeteners often do not know whether they are taking one or the other, or indeed a mixture of both. This review does not, therefore, consider them separately; however, when a distinction is made in a particular study, this is mentioned.

Case reports

Bladder cancer has been described in four persons who took artificial sweeteners; one took saccharin (4 tablets a day for many years)(Grasset, 1974), and three took cyclamates (Barkin et al., 1977). The latter persons consumed large daily doses of cyclamates, namely 75, 65 and 40-50 mg/kg bw, respectively [A dose of 50 mg/kg bw per day is equivalent to an intake by a 70 kg person of about seventy 50 mg tablets each day]. Two of these patients had diabetes mellitus and two were smokers.

Trends in bladder cancer (Table 1A)[1]

Burbank & Fraumeni (1970) examined bladder cancer death rates in the US for the years 1950-1967. There was no clear-cut break in the continuity of the trends in the age-specific or age-adjusted rates following the widespread introduction of artificial sweeteners (mainly a 10:1 mixture of cyclamate:saccharin) in 1962. There was also no break in the continuity of incidence trends for bladder cancer in Connecticut and New York states.

Armstrong & Doll (1974) carried out a cohort analysis of bladder cancer mortality in England and Wales for the period 1911-1970. This showed 'no evidence of any break in the continuity of the trends in either men or women which corresponds to the introduction of saccharin'.

[While these studies indicate that no marked increase in incidence of bladder cancer has occurred in the US and the UK following the increased use of artificial sweeteners, studies of

---

[1] The Working Group was aware of a study in progress in which information was being collected on patients with urinary bladder cancer, in particular on occupational exposure, geographical factors and eating habits (e.g., consumption of saccharin and cyclamates) (IARC, 1979).

incidence or mortality trends in populations are likely to be insensitive for three reasons: (1) the proportion of the population exposed to large amounts of artificial sweeteners is small. Therefore, unless there was an excess risk for humans of much higher magnitude than that suggested by experimental work in animals, only a small proportion of bladder cancers in the general population would be attributable to this exposure; (2) changes over time in the exposure of the general population to other risk factors, such as smoking and occupation, would also affect the rates; (3) early diagnosis or improvements in medical treatment or both, which have led to increased survival among patients with bladder cancer, mean that an increase in incidence may not be reflected in an increase in mortality].

Studies of patients with diabetes mellitus (Table 1B)

Kessler (1970) reported on the mortality experience of 21,447 diabetic patients registered at one diabetes clinic in Boston from 1930-1956, who were followed up until the end of 1959. Expected deaths were computed on the basis of the mortality of the population of Massachusetts. Bladder cancer mortality was less than expected in both sexes [for males: observed to expected deaths (O/E) = 14/18.09, Standardized Mortality Ratio (SMR) = 0.77, $P > 0.3$; for females: O/E = 7/11.52, SMR = 0.61, $P > 0.1$]. Respiratory cancer deaths were significantly lower in males (O/E = 46/71.7, SMR = 0.64, $P < 0.005$), a finding which may be only partly explained by the reduced cigarette consumption among diabetic men compared to men in the general population, since males also had lower than expected mortality for cancers other than those of the respiratory tract (O/E = 312/348.78, SMR = 0.89, $P < 0.05$). Females did not show a similar effect for either respiratory cancer (O/E = 25/19.7, SMR = 1.27, $P > 0.2$) or other cancers (O/E = 519/509.81, SMR = 1.01, $P > 0.5$) [There were some differences between the study and control populations (other than the presence of diabetes) which might have affected the results of the study. For instance, 17% of the diabetic group were Jews, compared with only 5% of the Massachusetts population. The study did not measure artificial sweetener consumption in diabetics and did not consider the possible role of sweeteners in the etiology of cancer].

Armstrong & Doll (1975) performed a case-control study using death certificates from England and Wales for the period 1966-1972: 18,733 persons with bladder cancer as the underlying cause of death constituted the cases, and a random sample of 19,709 persons with other cancers as the cause of death were used as controls. Among cases, diabetes mellitus was mentioned on the death certificates of 138 men and 81 women; the corresponding figures in controls (excluding cancer of the lung and pancreas) were 103 and 172. The relative risk of bladder cancer for male and female diabetics combined was 0.98, with 95% confidence limits of 0.70-1.38. Among a sample of 269 patients who died in 1971-1972 and who were chosen to determine the date of diagnosis from medical records, there was no increase in risk of bladder cancer in those who had had diabetes of long duration. An indication of saccharin consumption among diabetics was ascertained from a sample of 200 diabetics currently attending a diabetes clinic in Oxford and 200 controls matched by age and sex currently on the lists of the same general practices as the diabetics. These diabetics were shown to consume substantially more saccharin than the nondiabetic controls, and the duration of regular saccharin use by diabetics was highly correlated with the duration of the diabetes.

Armstrong *et al.* (1976) reported on the mortality experience of 5971 diabetics who were mainly new members of the British Diabetic Association from November 1965 until the end of 1968 and who were followed for 5-8 years to mid-1973. Expected deaths from bladder cancer and SMRs in the cohort of diabetics were calculated by comparison with the mortality experience of the population of England and Wales of comparable age and sex. Deaths from bladder cancer were fewer than expected: O/E = 4/5.8, SMR = 0.70 (not significant). Smoking-related cancers (i.e., those of buccal cavity and pharynx, oesophagus, respiratory system and bladder) were also less frequent - O/E = 30/61.1, SMR = 0.49, P< 0.01 - as was non-smoking related cancer - O/E = 98/107.0, SMR = 0.92 (not significant). Deaths from all cancers (128 observed) were significantly fewer than expected (168) (SMR = 0.76, P < 0.01). Data on saccharin consumption was gathered from a questionnaire sent to 4000 members of the British Diabetic Association (about 10% of the total membership) and returned by 77%: more than half of them used saccharin tablets daily, with an overall daily intake of 3-6 tablets, depending on age and sex; older men consumed more. Information relating to a sample of 61 survivors from the mortality study (100 were sent questionnaires) indicated that by the end of follow-up 10% (6) would have taken saccharin daily for 25 years or more, a further 13% (8) for between 10 and 25 years and 77% (47) for less than 10 years or not at all.

[The risk of bladder cancer in diabetics who do not use artificial sweeteners may be lower than that in the general population, either because of metabolic differences or differences in, say, their diet, use of drugs, exposure to tobacco or occupational factors. Therefore, derivation of an expectation from the general population for the risk of bladder cancer in diabetic populations may conceal a risk. The studies of diabetics cannot therefore be regarded as providing strong evidence for a lack of a carcinogenic effect of artificial sweeteners in humans. These studies of diabetic patients are the only ones that have investigated the possible carcinogenic effect on organs other than the bladder, and, so far, there is no evidence for such an effect].

Case-control studies

Table 2 summarizes in chronological sequence of publication the 7 case-control studies of bladder cancer available to the Working Group in which subjects were asked how much artificial sweetener they used. These studies will be considered in turn.

Morgan & Jain (1974) reported a study in which histologically confirmed cases of transitional-cell carcinoma of the urinary bladder were individually matched to a control patient according to age and sex. Male controls had benign prostatic hypertrophy, while female controls had stress incontinence. Rates of response to a mailed questionnaire were:

TABLE 1. Epidemiological studies relating to use of artificial sweeteners and bladder cancer

A. Studies of trends in bladder cancer

Reference	Data	Results
Burbank & Fraumeni (1970)	US bladder cancer deaths, 1950-1967; US total cyclamate-saccharin consumption, 1950-1969	No clear-cut increase since widespread introduction of artificial sweeteners
Armstrong & Doll (1974)	UK bladder cancer deaths, 1911-1970; UK per caput saccharin consumption, 1939-1972	No evidence of break in trends corresponding to increased saccharin use

B. Studies of patients with diabetes mellitus

Reference	Years	Populations	Relative risk (RR) & standardized mortality ratio (SMR) of bladder cancer	Significance (95% confidence interval)
Kessler (1970)	1930-1956 (registration); 1931-1959 (follow-up)	Observed: 14 male and 7 female bladder cancer deaths among 21,447 diabetics at outpatient clinic. Expected: from age/sex specific rates in Massachusetts over the same period	(m) SMR = 0.8; (f) SMR = 0.6	P>0.3; P>0.1

Table 1 (contd)

Reference	Years	Populations	Relative risk (RR) & standardized mortality ratio (SMR) of bladder cancer	Significance (95% confidence interval)
Armstrong & Doll (1975)	1966-1972	*Observed*: 138 males and 81 females with diabetes mentioned on death certificate out of 18,773 persons who died of bladder cancer in the UK *Expected*: proportion with mention of diabetes in pooled observations of bladder cancer (18,733) and other cancer deaths (not lung or pancreas) (19,709)	(m) RR = 1.00 (f) RR = 0.97	(0.6 - 1.6) (0.6 - 1.6)
Armstrong *et al.* (1976)	1965-1968 (registration) 1965-1973 (follow-up)	*Observed*: 4 bladder cancer deaths among 1207 total deaths in 5971 UK diabetics followed prospectively for 5-8 years *Expected*: from 10% random sample of all deaths in UK, 1972, for similar age/sex	SMR = 0.7	not significant (0.19 - 1.79)

TABLE 2. Summary of case-control studies of bladder cancer in relation to the use of artificial sweeteners

Reference	Years subjects recruited	No. of subjects		Source of information on artificial sweetener consumption
		Cases	Controls	
Morgan & Jain (1974)	Not stated	(m) 158 (f) 74	158 74	MQ
Simon et al. (1975)	1965-1971	(f) 135	390	MQ
Howe et al. (1977)	1974-1976	(m) 480 (f) 152	480 152	PI
Wynder & Goldsmith (1977)	1969-1974	(m) 132 (f) 31	124 29	PI
Miller et al. (1978)	Not stated	(m) 188 (f) 77	376 154	SQ
Connolly et al. (1978)	Not stated	(m) 243 (f) 98	479 194	NK
Kessler & Clark (1978)	1972-1975	(m) 365 (f) 154	365 154	PI

m - male
f - female
MQ - mailed questionnaire
PI - personal interview
SQ - supervised questionnaire
NK - not known
NS - not statistically significant

Table 2 (contd)

Source of subjects	Relative risk (95% confidence interval)	Matching variables
Not stated Controls had benign prostatic hypertrophy (m) and stress incontinence (f)	1.00^a $(0.6\text{-}1.8)^f$ 0.35^a $(0.1\text{-}0.8)^f$	Sex, age ($\pm$ 5 yrs)
White subjects from 10 hospitals Controls without urinary problems from same hospitals	Cyclamate 1.2^b $(0.5\text{-}2.6)$ Saccharin 1.0^b $(0.5\text{-}1.7)$	Age ($\pm$ 4 yrs), urban/rural, discharge date
All incident bladder cancer cases in 3 provinces in Canada Neighbourhood controls	1.6^c $(1.1\text{-}2.3)$ 1.6^c $(0.3\text{-}1.1)^f$	Sex, age ($\pm$ 5 yrs)
Bladder cancer patients from 17 hospitals Controls without 'tobacco-related disease'	0.7^c $(0.2\text{-}2.2)$ 0.7^c $(0.1\text{-}15)$	Sex, race, hospital status, age ($\pm$ 5 yrs)
All patients over 40 years at urology clinic: cases, bladder cancer; controls, all others	1.1^b (NS) 0.9^b (NS)	Sex, age ($\pm$ 5 yrs)
Not stated	0.9^d $(0.6\text{-}1.4)^f$ 0.7^d $(0.4\text{-}1.3)^f$	Sex, age ($\pm$ 5 yrs), residence
All bladder cancer patients in 19 hospitals Controls in same hospital cancer-free, no bladder complaints	1.1^e $(0.8\text{-}1.6)$ 0.8^e $(0.5\text{-}1.4)$	Sex, race, age ($\pm$ 3 yrs), marital status

[a] Prolonged regular use *versus* never use

[b] Usual adult use *versus* never use

[c] Ever use *versus* never use

[d] Extent of use not specified

[e] Use for 6 months or more *versus* never use; relative risk adjusted for many variables, including smoking, occupation, diabetes

[f] Confidence intervals not given in the published paper but calculated by the Working Group (approximate intervals for the ratio of discordant pairs in matched studies, or calculated using the method of Miettinen, 1969, 1970)

male cases, 67% and male controls, 57%; female cases, 73% and female controls, 57%. The actual analysis was based on 158 matched male case-control pairs and 74 matched female pairs. Data relating to 2 cases (1%) and 18 controls (10%) in men, and 17 cases (18%) and 17 controls (18%) in women could not be analysed due to lack of a suitable match. Prolonged regular use of any artificial sweetener was associated with a relative risk of 1.00 (not significant) in males and 0.35 (P <0.01) in females [The distribution of amount, frequency and duration of artificial sweetener consumption were not given, and the method of ascertaining the cases was not specified. It is not clear how many of the nonascertained subjects and those who were sent questionnaires had already died and to what extent the study was therefore one of long-term survivors of bladder cancer. The controls had diseases the treatment of which may have affected fluid intake, although this was not medically prescribed, and thus their intake of artificial sweeteners may also have been affected. For example, control women may have drunk less to reduce stress incontinence. On the other hand, women with stress incontinence might be more likely to be obese than cases and thus have a higher consumption of artificial sweeteners].

From pathology records and the diagnostic indices of 10 hospitals in Massachusetts (other than Boston) and Rhode Island, Simon et al. (1975) identified 216 white women in whom lower urinary tract cancer (95% of which were bladder cancer) was diagnosed between 1965 and 1971. Three female controls without urinary tract problems were matched to each case according to race, age (± 5 years), place of residence (urban/rural) and hospital. Forty of the cases were found to have died and 77% of the remainder responded to a mail questionnaire, leaving 135 cases for analysis. The corresponding response rate among controls was 72%. Neither saccharin (RR, 1.0) nor cyclamate (RR, 1.2) were significantly associated with lower urinary tract cancer. The absence of such an effect was demonstrated in tea- as well as coffee-drinkers [No data were presented on the possible risk of cancer in relation to amount, frequency or duration of artificial sweetener use].

A study by Howe et al. (1977) is the only one that reported a positive association between artificial sweetener use and bladder cancer. Cases were derived from all nonrecurrent, newly-diagnosed bladder cancer patients in 3 Canadian provinces between April 1974 and June 1976. They were identified through population-based tumour registries, pathologists and urologists. Out of 821 eligible cases, 56 were dead, 65 refused to be interviewed, 25 were too ill and 34 were not approached because their doctors did not want their patients to be interviewed, thus leaving 641. The final analysis was actually based on 632 cases (480 men and 152 women), representing 77% of all the eligible cases. The cases were interviewed in their homes, and controls were sought by approaching neighbours who lived a specified number of homes away from the case and continuing from one home to another until a control of the same sex and age (within 5 years) was found. A statistically significant excess of artificial sweetener use was reported in male cases (RR, 1.6); and this excess was also present when the analysis was restricted to the 82% of men who used artificial sweeteners that contained only saccharin. The relative risks of bladder cancer in male users of these brands (relative to those in men who had never consumed saccharin) were 1.5 and 2.1 among men who consumed less than 2500 and 2500 or more saccharin tablets per year, respectively.

Similarly, the relative risks were 1.4 and 2.0 among men who used such saccharin tablets for less than 3 years and more than 3 years, respectively. The trends in both associations were statistically significant (P=0.02, P=0.03). The risk of bladder cancer was lower among female users of artificial sweeteners than among women who never used them (RR, 0.6; 95% confidence interval, 0.3-1.1). The possible confounding effects of smoking and coffee consumption on the risk of bladder cancer were analysed after discarding pairs discordant with respect to smoking or coffee consumption, using the following groupings: ≤10,000 and >10,000 packs of cigarettes lifetime consumption and 'never' and 'ever' instant coffee consumption [This analysis for confounding was described as inadequate in a *Lancet* editorial article (Anon., 1977), and the study was thus considered to be inconclusive].

In response to the *Lancet* editorial, Miller & Howe (1977) presented further analyses relating to men to better control for smoking and coffee consumption. This analysis was unmatched. When instant coffee consumption was considered in three groups (none, <1½ cups per day and ≥1½ cups per day), the relative risk for each group and the summary relative risk remained unchanged, at 1.6 [95% confidence interval, 1.1-2.4]. The authors also divided cigarette consumption into 5 groups, namely: none (RR, 0.7), former smokers of <5000 packs lifetime consumption (1.5), former smokers of ≥5000 packs lifetime consumption (2.1), current smokers of <15 cigarettes/day (1.0) and current smokers of ≥15 cigarettes/ day (1.7). The summary relative risk was given as 1.7 (P=0.01, one-tailed); but this excluded data relating to nonsmokers [Inclusion of the latter lowered the summary relative risk estimate to 1.5 (P=0.03, one-tailed; 95% confidence interval, 1.0-2.3].

Howe *et al*. (1979) have also analysed their data on men using a logistic regression analysis which took account of the case-control matching. Cigarette consumption was related to both artificial sweetener use and bladder cancer and was the principal confounding variable. When the confounding variables (life-time tobacco consumption, 'high risk' occupations, use of non-public water supply, bladder infection, diabetes, school marks, lifetime aspirin use, daily coffee use) were controlled for simultaneously, the relative risk of bladder cancer in relation to artificial sweetener consumption (divided into 5 groups) was as follows:

Artificial sweetener consumption (tablets/day)	Relative risk (95% confidence interval)
0	1.0
1-4	0.9 (0.4-2.1)
5-6	1.6 (0.6-4.3)
7-8	1.1 (0.3-4.0)
9 or more	2.8 (0.9-8.9)

The authors reported that when artificial sweetener use was considered as a continuous variable, the overall linear trend is statistically significant using a one-tailed test (P=0.03) [This implies that the trend is not likely to be statistically significant at the conventional level of P=0.05 if a two-tailed test were used].

When the analysis was restricted to those individuals who reported using saccharin alone, the results were similar. The relative risk estimates for up to 4, 4-8, and more than 8 tablets of saccharin per day were: 0.9, 1.4 and 3.1 (Howe et al., 1979) [The Working Group noted that the confidence limits were not reported].

[The numbers of men in each artificial sweetener consumption group are not given in the paper; however, the Working Group inferred, on the basis of the width of the reported confidence intervals (see table above), that they were small. While the data are consistent with no effect of artificial sweetener use on the risk of bladder cancer, there remains a suspicion of such an effect among heavy users of artificial sweeteners. An unknown number of eligible neighbourhood controls who were not at home when the interviewer visited could not be included in the study. It is possible that factors (e.g., social) influencing their absence were also related to saccharin consumption and so may have biassed the estimates of relative risk].

Wynder & Goldsmith (1977) studied bladder cancer patients and controls matched for sex, race, age and 'hospital status'. Thirteen of 132 male cases (10%) and 16 of 124 male controls (13%) used artificial sweeteners (RR, 0.7; not significant). The comparable data for females were 4 of 31 cases (13%) and 5 of 29 controls (17%) (RR, 0.7; not significant) [It was not clearly stated whether each case-control pair came from the same hospital; the subjects were recruited from 17 hospitals throughout the USA].

Miller et al. (1978) studied 265 patients with bladder cancer and 530 matched controls (two for each case) matched for sex and age (± 5 years). All subjects were registered as outpatients at a Canadian urology clinic. Data were collected using a self-administered questionnaire supervised by clinic staff [The diagnosis was unknown to both patient and staff at the time the data were collected]. There was no significant risk associated with the regular use of artificial sweeteners (RR, 1.1 for men and 0.9 for women) [The diagnoses of controls are not given, and no account was taken of possible confounding factors, such as smoking].

Connolly et al. (1978) published a letter reporting no excess of artificial sweetener users in 341 patients with bladder cancer, compared with 673 controls matched for sex, age (± 5 years) and place of residence (county and urban/rural) [The relative risk was 0.93 for men and 0.70 for women. No information was provided on how the cases and controls were ascertained or on the distribution or effect of potential confounding variables. No data were presented on the extent, duration or length of exposure to artificial sweeteners].

Kessler & Clark (1978), expanding the work of Kessler (1976), ascertained all of 1300 histologically confirmed bladder cancer cases discharged from 19 Baltimore hospitals between 1972 and 1975. Of these, 519 (40%) (365 males, 154 females) were interviewed; the remainder consisted of subjects who died (509), those who were unable or refused to be interviewed (115) and those who were identified late (157). One control patient without a diagnosis of cancer and without a bladder condition was matched with each case on the basis of hospital, age (± 3 years), sex, race, date of admission and current marital status. Personal interviews were used to obtain information on the use of foods and beverages containing artificial sweeteners by frequency, quantity, duration and brand name. Use of saccharin or cyclamates during the year prior to the cancer diagnosis was ignored for each case and matched control. Matched-pair analysis of relative risks for those using any form of artificial sweeteners 'more than occasionally' were 0.97 for men (95% confidence limits, 0.70-1.35), 1.00 (0.63-1.59) for women and 0.98 (0.75-1.28) overall. Adjustment of these figures for such potential confounding factors as smoking, occupation, obesity and diabetes yielded relative risks of 1.11 (0.78-1.58) for men, 0.80 (0.47-1.39) for women and 1.04 (0.80-1.40) overall in users of 6 months' duration or more. No evidence of a dose-response trend was obtained for either sex when users were subdivided into three equal groups according to lifetime exposure. Relative risks calculated separately for saccharin were 1.08 (0.79-1.48) for men and 0.87 (0.55-1.37) for women; for cyclamates these figures were 1.12 (0.79-1.58) and 0.74 (0.46-1.19) [These results make a relative risk of about 1.5 or higher unlikely, but they are not inconsistent with a relative risk closer to 1. Restriction of the cases to survivors leaves open the possibility that use of artificial sweeteners might be higher in cases with rapidly lethal tumours, who would have been less likely to be interviewed].

[Neither Howe et al. (1977) nor Kessler & Clark (1978) found a statistically significant difference in the proportion of cases and controls who ate foods or drank beverages containing artificial sweeteners. However, intake of sweeteners from these sources may be of too short duration and involve too young an age group to allow detection of an effect].

General

Examination of time trends in the USA and in England and Wales shows that there has been no marked increase in the incidence of bladder cancer following the rapid increase in use of artificial sweeteners. In the UK, diabetics as a group consume higher quantities of artificial sweeteners than the general population and experience a lower mortality from bladder cancer than the general population. However, because of metabolic differences or differences in diet, use of drugs, exposure to tobacco or occupational factors in diabetics, this finding cannot exclude a carcinogenic effect of sweeteners.

Seven case-control studies were considered by the Working Group. Five were negative but were limited by some inadequacies in experimental design. Only two examined possible confounding factors in detail. Of these, one suggested that artificial sweetener use was positively associated with bladder cancer in men but not in women. The association was limited to men who used nine or more tablets of artificial sweeteners per day or if only saccharin was considered, who consumed an average of more than eight tablets of saccharin per day; the relative risk in both instances was about 3. However, in these small groups, the result could have been due to chance, to confounding factors that were not included in the analysis, or (as in any study with relative risks near 1) to residual effects of those confounding factors that were considered in the analysis.

In 6 out of the 7 case-control studies reviewed, women with bladder cancer took less artificial sweeteners than the controls, and in one study this difference was statistically significant. This observation provides no evidence that artificial sweeteners cause bladder cancer in women.

The epidemiological data taken as a whole cannot with confidence exclude a small increase in risk but provide no clear evidence that artificial sweeteners cause bladder cancer in humans.

Footnote

After the meeting of the Working Group, two epidemiological investigations (Morrison & Buring, 1980; Wynder & Stellman, 1980) were reported.

The study by Morrison & Buring evaluated the relation between cancer of the lower urinary tract and the use of artificial sweeteners in a case-control study of 592 patients with lower-urinary-tract cancer (94 per cent of whom had a bladder tumour) and 536 controls chosen from the general population of the study area. A history of use of artificial sweeteners and exposure to other known or suspected risk factors was determined by interview. In those who had used dietetic beverages and in those who had used sugar substitutes, the relative risk of lower-urinary-tract cancer was estimated as 0.9 (0.7 to 1.2, 95% confidence interval), as compared with 1 in nonusers of artificial sweeteners. Among men, the relative risk was 0.8 (0.6 to 1.1) in those who had used dietetic beverages and 0.8 (0.5 to 1.1) in those who had used sugar substitutes. Among women, the corresponding relative risks were 1.6 (0.9 to 2.7) and 1.5 (0.9 to 2.6). Increasing frequency or duration of use of artificial sweeteners was not consistently associated with increasing relative risk. This study suggests that, as a group, users of artificial sweeteners have little or no excess risk of cancer of the lower urinary tract [Authors' summary].

The study by Wynder & Stellman was a case-control study of 302 men and 65 women with bladder cancer and an equal number of controls matched for age, sex, hospital and hospital-room status. No association was found between the use of artificial sweeteners or diet-beverage consumption and bladder cancer. The relative risk of bladder cancer (95% confidence interval) among men was 0.9 (0.7-1.3) for artificial sweetener use and 0.8 (0.6-1.2) for diet-beverage consumption; among women, the relative risks were 0.6 (0.3-1.4) and 0.6 (0.3-1.3), respectively. These relative risk estimates did not vary appreciably when a number of potential confounding variables were controlled for, namely, history of diabetes, obesity, occupation, education, religion and coffee or tea consumption. No dose-response relationships between consumption of artificial sweeteners or diet beverages and quantity or duration of use were observed.

References

Anon. (1977) Bladder cancer and saccharin. *Lancet, ii*, 592-593

Armstrong, B. & Doll, R. (1974) Bladder cancer mortality in England and Wales in relation to cigarette smoking and saccharin consumption. *Br. J. prev. soc. Med., 28*, 233-240

Armstrong, B. & Doll, R. (1975) Bladder cancer mortality in diabetics in relation to saccharin consumption and smoking habits. *Br. J. prev. soc. Med., 29*, 73-81

Armstrong B., Lea, A.J., Adelstein, A.M., Donovan, J.W., White, G.C. & Ruttle, S. (1976) Cancer mortality and saccharin consumption in diabetics. *Br. J. prev. soc. Med., 30*, 151-157

Barkin, M., Comisarow, R.H., Taranger, L.A. & Canada, A. (1977) Three cases of human bladder cancer following high dose cyclamate ingestion. *J. Urol., 118*, 258-259

Burbank, F. & Fraumeni, J.F., Jr (1970) Synthetic sweetener consumption and bladder cancer trends in the United States. *Nature, 227*, 296-297

Connolly, J.G., Rider, W.D., Rosenbaum, L. & Chapman, J.-A. (1978) Relation between the use of artificial sweeteners and bladder cancer. *Can. med. Assoc. J., 119*, 408

Grasset, A.V. (1974) Saccharin and carcinoma of the bladder. *Can. med. Assoc. J., 110*, 1135,1137

Howe, G.R., Burch, J.D., Miller, A.B., Morrison, B., Gordon, P., Weldon, L., Chambers, L.W., Fodor, G. & Winsor, G.M. (1977) Artificial sweeteners and human bladder cancer. *Lancet, ii*, 578-581

Howe, G.R., Burch, J.D., Miller, A.B., Cook, G.M., Esteve, J., Morrison, B., Gordon, P., Chambers, L.W., Fodor, G. & Winsor, G.M. (1979) Tobacco use, occupation, coffee, various nutrients, and bladder cancer. *J. natl Cancer Inst.* (in press)

IARC (1979) *Directory of On-Going Research in Cancer Epidemiology, 1979 (IARC Scientific Publications No. 28)*, Lyon, Abstract no. 203, p. 108

Kessler, I.I. (1970) Cancer mortality among diabetics. *J. natl Cancer Inst., 44*, 673-686

Kessler, I.I. (1976) Non-nutritive sweeteners and human bladder cancer: preliminary findings. *J. Urol., 115*, 143-146

Kessler, I.I. & Clark, J.P. (1978) Saccharin, cyclamate, and human bladder cancer. No evidence of an association. *J. Am. med. Assoc., 240*, 349-355

Miettinen, O.S. (1969) Individual matching with multiple controls in the case of all-or-none response. *Biometrics, 25*, 339-355

Miettinen, O.S. (1970) Estimation of relative risk from individually matched series. *Biometrics, 26*, 75-86

Miller, A.B. & Howe, G.R. (1977) Artificial sweeteners and bladder cancer. *Lancet, ii*, 1221-1222

Miller, C.T., Neutel, C.I., Nair, R.C., Marrett, L.D., Last, J.M. & Collins, W.E. (1978) Relative importance of risk factors in bladder carcinogenesis. *J. chron. Dis., 31*, 51-56

Morgan, R.W. & Jain, M.G. (1974) Bladder cancer: smoking, beverages and artificial sweeteners. *Can. med. Assoc. J., 111*, 1067-1070

Morrison, A.S. & Buring, J.E. (1980) Artificial sweeteners and cancer of the lower urinary tract. *New Engl. J. Med., 302,* 537-541

Simon, D., Yen, S. & Cole, P. (1975) Coffee drinking and cancer of the lower urinary tract. *J. natl Cancer Inst., 54*, 587-591

Wynder, E.L. & Goldsmith, R. (1977) The epidemiology of bladder cancer. A second look. *Cancer, 40*, 1246-1268

Wynder, E.L. & Stellman, S.D. (1980) Artificial sweetener use and bladder cancer: a case control study. *Science* (in press)

SUPPLEMENTARY CORRIGENDA TO VOLUMES 1-21

Volume 4
p. 90   *(c)* last line   *replace* 'mg' *by* 'ng'

CUMULATIVE INDEX TO IARC MONOGRAPHS ON THE EVALUATION

OF THE CARCINOGENIC RISK OF CHEMICALS TO HUMANS

Numbers in bold indicate volume, and numbers in italics indicate page. References to corrigenda are given in parentheses. Compounds marked with an asterisk (*) were considered by the Working Groups, but monographs were not prepared because adequate data on their carcinogenicity were not available.

B

C

| Sudan red 7B | **8**, *253* | |
| Sunset yellow FCF | **8**, *257* | |

T

2,4,5-T and esters	**15**, *273*	
Tannic acid	**10**, *253*	(corr, **16**, *387*)
Tannins	**10**, *254*	
Terephthalic acid*		
Terpene polychlorinates (Strobane®)	**5**, *219*	
Testosterone	**6**, *209*	
	21, *519*	
Testosterone oenanthate	**21**, *521*	
Testosterone propionate	**21**, *522*	
1,1,2,2-Tetrachloroethane	**20**, *477*	
Tetrachloroethylene	**20**, *491*	
Tetraethyllead	**2**, *150*	
Tetrafluoroethylene	**19**, *285*	
Tetramethyllead	**2**, *150*	
Thioacetamide	**7**, *77*	
4,4'-Thiodianiline	**16**, *343*	
Thiouracil	**7**, *85*	
Thiourea	**7**, *95*	
Thiram	**12**, *225*	
2,4-Toluene diisocyanate	**19**, *303*	
2,6-Toluene diisocyanate	**19**, *303*	
ortho-Toluenesulphonamide	**22**, *121*	
ortho-Toluidine and its hydrochloride	**16**, *349*	
Toxaphene (polychlorinated camphenes)	**20**, *327*	
1,1,1-Trichloroethane	**20**, *515*	
1,1,2-Trichloroethane	**20**, *533*	
Trichloroethylene	**11**, *263*	
	20, *545*	
2,4,5- and 2,4,6-Trichlorophenols	**20**, *349*	

IARC MONOGRAPHS ON THE EVALUATION
OF THE CARCINOGENIC RISK OF CHEMICALS TO HUMANS

IARC Publications continued on inside back cover

IARC SCIENTIFIC PUBLICATIONS

WHO/IARC publications may be obtained, direct or through booksellers, from:

ALGERIA: Société Nationale d'Edition et de Diffusion, 3 bd Zirout Youcef, ALGIERS

ARGENTINA: Carlos Hirsch SRL, Florida 165, Galerias Güemes, Escritorio 453/465, BUENOS AIRES

AUSTRALIA: *Mail Order Sales:* Australian Government Publishing Service, P.O. Box 84, CANBERRA A.C.T. 2600; *or over the counter from* Australian Government Publishing Service Bookshops *at:* 70 Alinga Street, CANBERRA CITY A.C.T. 2600; 294 Adelaide Street, BRISBANE, Queensland 4000; 347 Swanston Street, MELBOURNE, VIC 3000; 309 Pitt Street, SYDNEY, N.S.W. 2000; Mt Newman House, 200 St. George's Terrace, PERTH, WA 6000; Industry House, 12 Pirie Street, ADELAIDE, SA 5000; 156–162 Macquarie Street, HOBART, TAS 7000 — Hunter Publications, 58A Gipps Street, COLLINGWOOD, VIC 3066

AUSTRIA: Gerold & Co., Graben 31, 1011 VIENNA I

BANGLADESH: The WHO Programme Coordinator, G.P.O. Box 250, DACCA 5 — The Association of Voluntary Agencies, P.O. Box 5045, DACCA 5

BELGIUM: Office international de Librairie, 30 avenue Marnix, 1050 BRUSSELS — *Subscriptions to World Health only:* Jean de Lannoy, 202 avenue du Roi, 1060 BRUSSELS

BRAZIL: Biblioteca Regional de Medicina OMS/OPS, Unidade de Venda de Publicações, Caixa Postal 20.381, Vila Clementino, 04023 SÃO PAULO, S.P.

BURMA: *see* India, WHO Regional Office

CANADA: *Single and bulk copies of individual publications (not subscriptions):* Canadian Public Health Association, 1335 Carling Avenue, Suite 210, OTTAWA, Ont. K1Z 8N8. *Subscriptions: Subscription orders, accompanied by cheque made out to the* Royal Bank of Canada, OTTAWA, Account World Health Organization, *should be sent to the* World Health Organization, P.O. Box 1800, Postal Station B, OTTAWA, Ont. K1P 5R5. *Correspondence concerning subscriptions should be addressed to the* World Health Organization, Distribution and Sales, 1211 GENEVA 27, Switzerland.

CHINA: China National Publications Import Corporation, P.O. Box 88, BEIJING (PEKING)

COLOMBIA: Distrilibros Ltd, Pío Alfonso García, Carrera 4a, Nos 36–119, CARTAGENA

CYPRUS: Publishers' Distributors Cyprus, 30 Democratias Ave Ayios Dhometious, P.O. Box 4165, NICOSIA

CZECHOSLOVAKIA: Artia, Ve Smeckach 30, 111 27 PRAGUE 1

DENMARK: Munksgaard Ltd, Norregade 6, 1165 COPENHAGEN K

ECUADOR: Libreria Científica S.A., P.O. Box 362, Luque 223, GUAYAQUIL

EGYPT: Nabaa El Fikr Bookshop, 55 Saad Zaghloul Street, ALEXANDRIA

EL SALVADOR: Libreria Estudiantil, Edificio Comercial B No 3, Avenida Libertad, SAN SALVADOR

FIJI: The WHO Programme Coordinator, P.O. Box 113, SUVA

FINLAND: Akateeminen Kirjakauppa, Keskuskatu 2, 00101 HELSINKI 10

FRANCE: Librairie Arnette, 2 rue Casimir-Delavigne, 75006 PARIS

GERMAN DEMOCRATIC REPUBLIC: Buchhaus Leipzig, Postfach 140, 701 LEIPZIG

GERMANY, FEDERAL REPUBLIC OF: Govi-Verlag GmbH, Ginnheimerstrasse 20, Postfach 5360, 6236 ESCHBORN — W. E. Saarbach, Postfach 101610, Follerstrasse 2, 5000 KÖLN 1 — Alex. Horn, Spiegelgasse 9, Postfach 3340, 6200 WIESBADEN

GHANA: Fides Enterprises, P.O. Box 1628, ACCRA

GREECE: G. C. Eleftheroudakis S.A., Librairie internationale, rue Nikis 4, ATHENS (T. 126)

HAITI: Max Bouchereau, Librairie "A la Caravelle", Boîte postale 111-B, PORT-AU-PRINCE

HONG KONG: Hong Kong Government Information Services, Beaconsfield House, 6th Floor, Queen's Road, Central, VICTORIA

HUNGARY: Kultura, P.O.B. 149, BUDAPEST 62 — Akadémiai Könyvesbolt, Váci utca 22, BUDAPEST V

ICELAND: Snaebjørn Jonsson & Co., P.O. Box 1131, Hafnarstraeti 9, REYKJAVIK

INDIA: WHO Regional Office for South-East Asia, World Health House, Indraprastha Estate, Ring Road, NEW DELHI 110002 — Oxford Book & Stationery Co., Scindia House, NEW DELHI 110001; 17 Park Street, CALCUTTA 700016 (*Sub-agent*)

INDONESIA: M/s Kalman Book Service Ltd, Jln. Cikini Raya No. 63, P.O. Box 3105/Jkt., JAKARTA

IRAN: Iranian Amalgamated Distribution Agency, 151 Khiaban Soraya, TEHERAN

IRAQ: Ministry of Information, National House for Publishing, Distributing and Advertising, BAGHDAD

IRELAND: The Stationery Office, DUBLIN 4

ISRAEL: Heiliger & Co., 3 Nathan Strauss Street, JERUSALEM

ITALY: Edizioni Minerva Medica, Corso Bramante 83–85, 10126 TURIN; Via Lamarmora 3, 20100 MILAN

JAPAN: Maruzen Co. Ltd, P.O. Box 5050, TOKYO International, 100–31

KOREA, REPUBLIC OF: The WHO Programme Coordinator, Central P.O. Box 540, SEOUL

KUWAIT: The Kuwait Bookshops Co. Ltd, Thunayan Al-Ghanem Bldg, P.O. Box 2942, KUWAIT

LAO PEOPLE'S DEMOCRATIC REPUBLIC: The WHO Programme Coordinator, P.O. Box 343, VIENTIANE

LEBANON: The Levant Distributors Co. S.A.R.L., Box 1181, Makdassi Street, Hanna Bldg, BEIRUT

LUXEMBOURG: Librairie du Centre, 49 bd Royal, LUXEMBOURG

MALAWI: Malawi Book Service, P.O. Box 30044, Chichiti, BLANTYRE 3

MALAYSIA: The WHO Programme Coordinator, Room 1004, Fitzpatrick Building, Jalan Raja Chulan, KUALA LUMPUR 05–02 — Jubilee (Book) Store Ltd, 97 Jalan Tuanku Abdul Rahman, P.O. Box 629, KUALA LUMPUR 01–08 — Parry's Book Center, K. L. Hilton Hotel, Jln. Treacher, P.O. Box 960, KUALA LUMPUR

MEXICO: La Prensa Médica Mexicana, Ediciones Científicas, Paseo de las Facultades 26, Apt. Postal 20–413, MEXICO CITY 20, D.F.

MONGOLIA: *see* India, WHO Regional Office

MOROCCO: Editions La Porte, 281 avenue Mohammed V, RABAT

MOZAMBIQUE: INLD, Caixa Postal 4030, MAPUTO

NEPAL: *see* India, WHO Regional Office

NETHERLANDS: N. V. Martinus Nijhoff's Boekhandel en Uitgevers Maatschappij, Lange Voorhout 9, THE HAGUE 2000

NEW ZEALAND: Government Printing Office, Mulgrave Street, Private Bag, WELLINGTON 1. *Government Bookshops at:* Rutland Street, P.O. 5344, AUCKLAND; 130 Oxford Terrace, P.O. Box 1721, CHRISTCHURCH; Alma Street, P.O. Box 857, HAMILTON; Princes Street, P.O. Box 1104, DUNEDIN — R. Hill & Son Ltd, Ideal House, Cnr Gillies Avenue & Eden St., Newmarket, AUCKLAND 1

NIGERIA: University Bookshop Nigeria Ltd, University of Ibadan, IBADAN — G. O. Odatuwa Publishers & Booksellers Co., 9 Benin Road, Okirigwe Junction, SAPELE, BENDEL STATE

NORWAY: J. G. Tanum A/S, P.O. Box 1177 Sentrum, OSLO 1

PAKISTAN: Mirza Book Agency, 65 Shahrah–E–Quaid–E–Azam, P.O. Box 729, LAHORE 3

PAPUA NEW GUINEA: The WHO Programme Coordinator, P.O. Box 5896, BOROKO

PHILIPPINES: World Health Organization, Regional Office for the Western Pacific, P.O. Box 2932, MANILA — The Modern Book Company Inc., P.O. Box 632, 926 Rizal Avenue, MANILA

POLAND: Składnica Księgarska, ul Mazowiecka 9, 00052 WARSAW (*except periodicals*) — BKWZ Ruch, ul Wronia 23, 00840 WARSAW (*periodicals only*)

PORTUGAL: Livraria Rodrigues, 186 Rua do Ouro, LISBON 2

SIERRA LEONE: Njala University College Bookshop (University of Sierra Leone), Private Mail Bag, FREETOWN

SINGAPORE: The WHO Programme Coordinator, 144 Moulmein Road, G.P.O. Box 3457, SINGAPORE 1 — Select Books (Pte) Ltd, 215 Tanglin Shopping Centre, 2/F, 19 Tanglin Road, SINGAPORE 10

SOUTH AFRICA: Van Schaik's Bookstore (Pty) Ltd, P.O. Box 724, 268 Church Street, PRETORIA 0001

SPAIN: Comercial Atheneum S.A., Consejo de Ciento 130–136, BARCELONA 15; General Moscardó 29, MADRID 20 — Libreria Diaz de Santos, Lagasca 95, MADRID 6; Balmes 417 y 419, BARCELONA 6

SRI LANKA: *see* India, WHO Regional Office

SWEDEN: Aktiebolaget C.E. Fritzes Kungl. Hovbokhandel, Regeringsgatan 12, 10327 STOCKHOLM

SWITZERLAND: Medizinischer Verlag Hans Huber, Länggass Strasse 76, 3012 BERN 9

SYRIAN ARAB REPUBLIC: M. Farras Kekhia, P.O. Box No. 5221, ALEPPO

THAILAND: *see* India, WHO Regional Office

TUNISIA: Société Tunisienne de Diffusion, 5 avenue de Carthage, TUNIS

TURKEY: Haset Kitapevi, 469 Istiklal Caddesi, Beyoglu, ISTANBUL

UNITED KINGDOM: H.M. Stationery Office: 49 High Holborn, LONDON WC1V 6HB; 13a Castle Street, EDINBURGH EH2 3AR; 41 The Hayes, CARDIFF CF1 1JW; 80 Chichester Street, BELFAST BT1 4JY; Brazennose Street, MANCHESTER M60 8AS; 258 Broad Street, BIRMINGHAM B1 2HE; Southey House, Wine Street, BRISTOL BS1 2BQ. *All mail orders should be sent to* P.O. Box 569, LONDON SE1 9NH

UNITED STATES OF AMERICA: *Single and bulk copies of individual publications (not subscriptions):* WHO Publications Centre USA, 49 Sheridan Avenue, ALBANY, N.Y. 12210. *Subscriptions: Subscription orders, accompanied by check made out to the* Chemical Bank, New York, Account World Health Organization, *should be sent to the* World Health Organization, P.O. Box 5284, Church Street Station, NEW YORK, N.Y. 10249. *Correspondence concerning subscriptions should be addressed to the* World Health Organization, Distribution and Sales, 1211 GENEVA 27, Switzerland. *Publications are also available from the* United Nations Bookshop, NEW YORK, N.Y. 10017 *(retail only), and single and bulk copies of individual* International Agency for Research on Cancer *publications (not subscriptions) may also be ordered from the* Franklin Institute Press, Benjamin Franklin Parkway, Philadelphia, PA 19103

USSR: *For readers in the USSR requiring Russian editions:* Komsomolskij prospekt 18, Medicinskaja Kniga, MOSCOW — *For readers outside the USSR requiring Russian editions:* Kuzneckij most 18, Meždunarodnaja Kniga, MOSCOW G-200

VENEZUELA: Editorial Interamericana de Venezuela C.A., Apartado 50.785, CARACAS 105 — Librería del Este, Apartado 60.337, CARACAS 106 — Librería Médica Paris, Apartado 60.681, CARACAS 106

YUGOSLAVIA: Jugoslovenska Knjiga, Terazije 27/II, 11000 BELGRADE

ZAIRE: Librairie universitaire, avenue de la Paix Nº 167, B.P. 1682, KINSHASA I

Special terms for developing countries are obtainable on application to the WHO Programme Coordinators or WHO Regional Offices listed above or to the World Health Organization, Distribution and Sales Service, 1211 Geneva 27, Switzerland. Orders from countries where sales agents have not yet been appointed may also be sent to the Geneva address, but must be paid for in pounds sterling, US dollars, or Swiss francs.

Price: Sw. fr. 25.— US$ 15.— Prices are subject to change without notice.

IARC/1/80